POLYAMORY IN THE TWENTY-FIRST CENTURY

POLYAMORY IN THE TWENTY-FIRST CENTURY

Love and Intimacy with Multiple Partners

Deborah Anapol

Rowman & Littlefield Publishers, Inc.
Lanham • Boulder • New York • Toronto • Plymouth, UK

Published by Rowman & Littlefield Publishers, Inc.
A wholly owned subsidiary of The Rowman & Littlefield Publishing Group, Inc.
4501 Forbes Boulevard, Suite 200, Lanham, Maryland 20706
http://www.rowmanlittlefield.com

Estover Road, Plymouth PL6 7PY, United Kingdom

British Library Cataloguing in Publication Information

Library of Congress Cataloging-in-Publication Data Available

Anapol, Deborah.
  Polyamory in the 21st century : love and intimacy with multiple partners /
Deborah Anapol.
     p. cm.
  Includes bibliographical references and index.
  ISBN 978-1-4422-0021-0 (cloth : alk. paper)—ISBN 978-1-4422-0023-4
(electronic)
  1. Non-monogamous relationships. 2. Sexual ethics. 3. Open marriage.
4. Homosexuality—Psychological aspects. I. Title. II. Title: Polyamory in
the twenty first century.
  HQ980.A536 2010
  306.84'23--dc22

                                                                2010014094

⊗™ The paper used in this publication meets the minimum requirements of
American National Standard for Information Sciences—Permanence of Paper
for Printed Library Materials, ANSI/NISO Z39.48-1992.
Manufactured in the United States of America.

Printed in the United States of America

For the Next Generations

CONTENTS

INTRODUCTION

I have always characterized my position on polyamory as pro-choice rather than antimonogamy, but after thirty years as a participant observer in this strange new world, it's more the case than ever that I really have no position on whether people in general "should" be monogamous or not. The fact is that it's extremely rare to find anyone who has had only one sexual partner for his or her entire life. These days, it's increasingly unusual to find anyone who has only had one "significant other" throughout his or her life. So the question is not so much whether to love more than one but rather whether it works better to have multiple partners sequentially or at the same time. There are definitely some people who are far better off taking it one at a time, and there are some situations that cry out for other possibilities. I'm continually amazed both by the ingenuity, courage, and vulnerability of people who have made their own bodies and hearts the center for an inquiry into the true nature of love and by the persistent self-deception, lack of integrity, and callousness that others justify by calling what they are doing polyamory.

My first teachers in the realm of conscious relationship, who happened to live in an extremely loving and functional group marriage, repeatedly cautioned me not to get caught up in the glamour of multipartner relating. The form of the relationship is not so important, they would say. The form can change at any time. What counts is allowing love to dictate the form rather than attempting to force love into whatever mold the mind has decided is right. It took me many years to fully understand the wisdom they were imparting, so I suppose it's not surprising that I've found that this concept is the hardest thing to get across to people. Polyamory is less about how many people you're having sex with, feeling love for, or both than it is about allowing love (not lust) to lead us into whatever form is appropriate. Lisa Diamond's concept of *sexual fluidity*, which is discussed in chapter 8, comes closer to the core of addressing what I was trying to convey when I first started writing about polyamory but that has often been overlooked both by those who apply the label *polyamorous* to themselves and by those who study or write about polyamory.

With a few notable exceptions, most authorities, whether their influence is spiritually based or scientifically based, still maintain that monogamy is superior to polyamory, or, in some cases they express the conviction that polyamory is simply unworkable. Often, there is a refusal to acknowledge polyamory as a viable option, and instead the entire discourse is framed as monogamy and infidelity. This kind of cultural bias has been dubbed *mononormativity* and is just beginning to be questioned by academic researchers. I admit that there have been times when I've been in the midst of a particularly challenging relationship dilemma when I've doubted the viability of multipartner relating myself, and I've watched many clients go through similar passages. I'm sure some monogamists also find themselves questioning whether monogamy is possible, although they are far more likely to find fault with themselves or their spouse than with the institution of marriage.

The main point is that it is not a question of whether it's possible to have one partner or two or many or none but rather a question of whether to allow love to lead and to surrender to the direction that love chooses rather than surrendering to cultural conditioning, unruly emotions, peer pressure, or social censure. I, for one, cannot imagine loving any other way.

The truth is that when love (and I don't mean lust, although this also applies to sexual desire) is freed from restrictions determined by law, by society, or by immature personalities, it very often veers from the monogamous standard our culture has sought, mostly unsuccessfully, to enforce. And so a practical discussion about polyamory inevitably ends up addressing the many startling aspects of multipartner or open relationships because it is this aspect of allowing love to lead that is unfamiliar and often difficult at first, as well as being sensationalist, intriguing, and sometimes dramatic.

This is not a how-to book, nor is it a manifesto for responsible nonmo-nogamy. Instead, it is a no-doubt flawed attempt to impartially convey some of what I've come to understand about the phenomenon now called polyamory. Having been involved in this world both personally and pro-fessionally over the past three decades, I like to think that I've gained an understanding and perspective that may be useful to others with less experience. Like everyone else, I was naive and poorly informed when I first became aware of alternatives to monogamy and the nuclear family in the early 1980s. As a result of my instrumental role in starting today's global polyamory movement, some people have idealized me and put me on a pedestal, while others have demonized, criticized, challenged, or os-tracized me.

For the past twenty-five years, I've led hundreds of seminars and coached thousands of individuals and partners all over the world who are struggling to reconcile conflicting urges toward monogamy and polyamory and who are seeking help in overcoming their jealousy. I've written books and ar-ticles, produced conferences, given countless media interviews, appeared on television, and cofounded a magazine. I've lived in both monogamous and open marriages, been part of the extended family of a group marriage and the "other woman" in the open relationships of several couples, and over the years evolved an intimate network of friends and lovers that is still deepening and expanding apart from my own involvement. I've also raised two children who are now adults and have two grandchildren. While I'm interested in men primarily romantically and erotically, I've had intimate friendships with women as well. I confess that pain and power games are major turn-offs for me personally, and while I can see the value some find in exploring bondage, discipline, and sadomasochism, at least for a limited time, it's not an area I know firsthand. Nor have I any direct experience of the world of gay men or transsexuals. Some readers may find my overview of today's global polyamory movement overly heterosexual or annoyingly vanilla, while others may find this departure from monogamous standards shocking. I make no apologies and mean no disrespect; I simply prefer to stick with those aspects of polyamory where I have confidence that the breadth and depth of my knowledge equals that of anyone alive today.

I'm convinced that the incidence of polyamory is far higher than anyone suspects because so many people keep their private lives private. It's still the case that most people who are willing to speak out about their poly-amorous lives or even stand up and be counted are activists. I often come into contact with people for reasons having nothing to do with polyamory or even sex or relationships for that matter, but when they find out that I've written books on polyamory and taught seminars, they share their secret lives with me. Others seek me out for help when their out-of-the-box relationships run into trouble because of my reputation as a relationship coach experienced with polyamory. These people seldom feel an affinity with the polyamorous community, may not even identify as polyamorous, and would certainly never consider talking to a journalist, not even anonymously. Consequently, the universe of people I've spoken to is somewhat different from that of investigators who've looked to the organized polyamorous community for information.

One of the reasons polyamory is at once appealing and threatening is that it brings to the forefront our cultural confusion about the interface between sex and love. In my first book, *Love without Limits*, which was published in 1992, I used the term *sexualove* to describe the integration of love and sex. However, we all know that sex can take place independently of love (even when we're talking about romantic or erotic love) and vice versa. Furthermore, most people who ponder these things discover that they're not entirely sure what the distinguishing features are for either sex or love. I've attempted to differentiate the qualities of love in my 2005 book *The Seven Natural Laws of Love*, but I find that, in practice, many people identifying as polyamorous are still confounding and compartmentalizing love and sex. While on the subject of sex, I feel it's important to acknowledge that, except for a very brief mention, I've not addressed the topic of "safe sex" in this book. It's an important subject that is worthy of greater consideration than is possible within the confines of this overview of polyamory; in fact, I feel that its relevance extends far beyond the world of polyamory. There are many books, articles, and websites devoted to this subject that can be easily accessed by those seeking either practical or scientific information.

In the 1980s, after the sometimes wild abandon and recklessness of the sexual revolution had died down and AIDS and campaigns for teenage abstinence took center stage, those who refused to retreat to monogamy tended to be a serious, introspective bunch. Eccentric, extraordinarily creative, intelligent or idealistic, and shaped by traumatic or unconventional childhoods, near-death experiences, and spiritual awakenings—in those days choosing nonmonogamy meant swimming upstream in a cultural context that had turned suddenly fearful and hostile to anything remotely associated with free love. Polyamory was not something the average man or woman in the street was likely to go along with simply because it was trendy as is now beginning to be the case. Yet even in those days, three or four people in the middle of nowhere might accidentally fall in love with each other and quietly set out to build a life together. Before global Internet access, Google, and the Web made networking easy, such people were isolated and often imagined that they were the only ones in the whole world who'd discovered that love can be shared with more than one significant other.

The idea that monogamy, which is freely and consciously chosen, is a totally different affair from monogamy, which is demanded as a condition for love or enforced by legal codes, religious strictures, financial considerations, or social pressure, has been put forth by a number of thoughtful individuals. Of course this is so, and while I am unconvinced as yet that this higher-level monogamy is superior to all other relationship forms, I don't know that it's not. Some therapists have suggested that multipartner relating prevents attachment.[1] In my experience, it doesn't. True, plenty of people use multipartner relating as a strategy to avoid attachment, consciously or unconsciously, but attachment is a powerful force that can override any mental argument or situational defense, except perhaps in people whose capacity for bonding is already impaired because they were prevented from bonding with nurturing caretakers in infancy.

I'm more inclined to see a diversity of relationship forms, all based on compassion, respect, integrity, and goodwill, as appropriate for different people at different times and in different places. However, I am fairly certain that only those who have first allowed themselves the freedom to explore a variety of sexual and intimate relationships are capable of completely embracing monogamy in a sustainable and responsible way.

I first became interested in polyamory in the early 1980s while working on a grassroots global education project originating in the United States called the Planetary Initiative for the World We Choose. Inspired by the United Nations, the Planetary Initiative was intended to make people around the world more proactive about the megacrisis facing humanity as we transition into the postmodern era. In his 2009 book *Global Shift*, Edmund Bourne describes it this way:

A worldview shift is part of a broader change that includes a far-reaching cultural, economic, and political restructuring of society. Such a shift happened in Europe during the Renaissance, and also much earlier in ancient

Greece. This time it is happening globally and, unlike the past, it may occur rapidly, over several decades rather than one or two centuries. . . . Such a shift has been developing over the past three decades and will continue to evolve through much of the twenty-first century. . . . The primary problem is that the current worldview promotes a separatism that has been encoded into many of our social and economic institutions. It has led individuals and groups to prioritize their needs over the good of the whole, to exploit others and the natural environment, and to disassociate their own well-being from that of the world around them. . . . However, there are cultural movements, scientific advances and new assumptions that have contributed to a broader understanding of who we are and what we are capable of becoming.[2]

I view polyamory as one of the cultural movements to which Bourne is referring. In the early 1980s, as is still often the case, sex, love, family, and intimate relationships were almost entirely left out of the conversation on sustainability, ecology, and consciousness in the United States. Zero population growth (ZPG) was given a nod but without much consideration of the implications for relationships or family life. While feminist writers had been critiquing monogamy and the nuclear family for decades, the only real integration I found of sexual relationships with the larger picture was in the work of renowned philosopher and astrologer Dane Rudhyar, who was born in Paris but spent most of his life in the United States. His 1971 book *Directives for New Life* addressed the central place of less rigidly constructed but still focused intimate relationships in the transition to a new society. The Planetary Initiative materials that had already been developed when I came on the scene included modules on alternative/renewable energy, transportation, architecture, health care, economics, education, and government, but the domestic domain was conspicuously absent except for the rather mechanistic approach to ZPG. Since sex and relationships happened to be my area of professional expertise, I took it on myself to start researching alternatives to monogamy and the nuclear family, seeking models for ways of relating that were more ethical and sustainable than those common in the twentieth century.

At that time, I was just completing my graduate work in clinical psychology at the University of Washington with a specialization in human sexuality and the psychology of women. I had chosen sex and intimacy for my professional focus because I had become convinced by that time that ending the war between the sexes was the crucial missing piece for sustainable peace between nations and that world peace was crucial to the very survival of humanity. Indigenous wisdom tells us that in making any decision, we must consider its consequences for the next seven generations. As the grandmother of two preschoolers, this consideration is now a very personal one.

Since I first began researching alternatives to monogamy and the nuclear family nearly three decades ago, I've been in communication with tens of thousands of people around the world about their experiences with polyamory. Many of these people attended my seminars or conferences I organized or spoke at; some have been coaching clients or read my books; a few are also researchers, activists, or academics; and some are personal friends, family, or lovers. I've been in contact with quite a few of these people for fifteen years or more. I've watched them fall in love, once or many times; add partners to existing relationships; form new relationships; struggle with jealousy or addictions; confront deaths and life-threatening illness, career changes, and geographic changes; marry, divorce, and remarry; get pregnant; and raise children and send these children off to college. I've watched them open their relationships and close them, come out of the closet, get religion, lose religion, become financially successful, and lose their life savings.

I've done my best to protect the confidentiality of these people as well as their families and loved ones while also relating accurately the essence of their words. I have changed names, dates, locations, and details of appearance, professions, and avocations. In some cases, I have blended the words and the histories of different people into composites while always endeavoring to keep the significant facts true to life. The only exception to this is people who are teachers and writers who are already totally "out of the closet" and so public with their lifestyle that I would hardly be infringing on their privacy to name them. In fact, they wish to be known to a wider audience and perhaps to correct mistaken impressions of their lifestyle as sometimes portrayed by the media.

In all honesty, after twenty-five years as a relationship coach, seminar leader, and participant observer in the polyamory community, I'm not at all sure that polyamory can fulfill its potential for sustainable intimacy, as I hoped when I subtitled my 1992 book *Love without Limits* the "Quest for Sustainable Intimate Relationships." Nevertheless, as the twenty-first century rolls on, it's increasingly apparent that lifelong monogamy is more myth than actuality and that the nuclear family is an endangered species. Now more than ever, it's essential that we release our attachments to conditioned beliefs about love, sex, intimacy, and commitment and be willing to discover and embrace whatever works. The one thing that is abundantly clear is that what works may not be the same for all people or even for the same person at different points in life. In addition, while the health and happiness of the adults who are struggling to create all kinds of relationships while honoring their innate sexuality under very challenging conditions is vital, it is the well-being of the next generations that is of greatest consequence.

1

WHAT IS POLYAMORY?

Polyamory is an invented word for a different kind of relationship. *Poly* comes from Greek and means "many." *Amory* comes from Latin and means "love." Mixing Greek and Latin roots in one word is against the traditional rules, but then so is loving more than one person at a time when it comes to romantic or erotic love.

The word *polyamory* was created in the late 1980s by Morning Glory and Oberon Zell. This couple, who have been married since 1974, continue to enjoy a deeply bonded open relationship that has morphed in many directions over the years, including a live-in triad lasting ten years and a six-person group marriage that recently dissolved after ten years.

The Zells did not invent the lifestyle, which has come to be known as polyamory, nor did I, though we are among a handful of pioneers who have mapped this new territory and thought deeply about its implications over the past thirty some years. I use the word *polyamory* to describe the whole range of lovestyles that arise from an understanding that love cannot be forced to flow or be prevented from flowing in any particular direction. Love, which is allowed to expand, often grows to include a number of people. But to me, polyamory has more to do with an internal attitude of letting love evolve without expectations or demands that it look a particular way than it does with the number of partners involved.

Few people would deny that there's been a significant shift in the way marriage and intimate relationships have evolved over the past few decades. Most observers agree that traditional marriage is floundering. While some couples still manage to thrive, they are in the minority. Rising divorce rates, declining marriage rates, and the skyrocketing incidence of infidelity on the one hand and sexless marriage on the other have many people concerned about their prospects for marital bliss and newly curious about alternatives.

More and more people find themselves facing the discovery that life-long monogamy is more of a mirage than a reality. At the same time, most experts on marriage, family, and sexuality continue to write and speak as if all extramarital sex falls into the category of infidelity. Sometimes it's acknowledged that an affair may inadvertently have a positive impact on a troubled marriage, but as far as the authorities are concerned, polyamory or consensual inclusive relationships do not exist. End of conversation. The losers are those adventurous souls struggling to make sense of their ever-changing relationships. We are all understandably confused by un-spoken and uncharted shifts in the ways we mate, but trying to deny this is happening will not help us adapt to the changes already under way, nor will it help us evolve new ways of relating that are truly appropriate for the twenty-first century.

It's often been noted that changes in belief systems frequently lag be-hind changes in behavior, and nowhere is this more evident that in the realm of erotic love. Meanwhile, people are voting with their search en-gines. Fueled by the power of the newly expanded Internet, the concept called polyamory has spread like wildfire. A recent Google search turned up over 1.8 million entries. In less than two decades, the use of and the meanings attributed to this newly invented word have taken on a life of their own. These days, polyamory has become a bit of a buzzword and often means different things to different people. So if you're perplexed by polyamory, you're not alone. Some people are still confusing *polyamory* with *polygamy*, which technically means to be married to more than one person, regardless of gender, but which has come to imply the patriarchal style of marriage in which a man has more than one wife while the women are monogamous with their shared husband.

The *Oxford Dictionary* defines polyamory as "(1) The fact of having simultaneous close emotional relationships with two or more other indi-viduals, viewed as an alternative to monogamy, esp. in regard to matters of sexual fidelity; (2) the custom or practice of engaging in multiple sexual relationships with the knowledge and consent of all partners concerned." These two alternate definitions are themselves a source of confusion for many. Jenna had the impression that polyamory refers to the "simultaneous close emotional relationships with two or more others" and, when she got involved with Gary, was intrigued by the prospect of exploring how this worked. But when Gary described himself as polyamorous, he had the second definition in mind and was intent on engaging in multiple sexual relationships regardless of the degree of emotional closeness. Neither was aware that they had very different expectations about their relationship, and both were shocked and dismayed when they discovered they were operating according to different game plans. Resentment toward the other for having a different agenda was quick to undermine their budding romance.

Considering how few people risk having any conversation at all with a prospective partner about their intentions around sexual exclusivity, it's not surprising that Jenna and Gary failed to recognize that they had different expectations about polyamory. They were headed in the right direction, but without some guidance, they didn't quite arrive where they wanted to go.

FORM VERSUS VALUES

Because so much of the discussion about polyamory has focused on the form of the relationship rather than the underlying values and belief systems, such misunderstandings are all too common. Two different relationships can look pretty much the same from the outside but will be experienced entirely differently from the inside, that is, by the people who are engaged in them.

For example, let's take two married heterosexual couples. Both couples married in their early thirties and have been together for ten years. One couple has the traditional "forsaking all others till death do us part" agreement, but neither partner is emotionally or sexually satisfied. Sheila's biological clock was ticking when she decided to marry Fred. He is a good provider and enthusiastic father but prefers golf to sexual intimacy and avoids conflict whenever possible. Sheila's increasing sexual frustration and loneliness soon had her fantasizing about having an affair, but she was afraid of ending up divorced. She gradually withdrew from Fred sexually and emotionally, and he immersed himself in his business. Superficially, they look like the perfect couple, but Sheila would leave in a heartbeat if it weren't for their two sons.

Gina and Eric met while working for the same company. They were attracted to each other but hesitant to get sexually involved in the fishbowl of the workplace. Instead, they developed a friendship and had many long conversations about life and love, discovering that they shared a passion for spiritual matters and personal autonomy as well as cooking, surfing, and mountain climbing. As Gina put it, "I don't want to hold my partner prisoner, and I don't want to be imprisoned either." When they finally transitioned from friendship to romance, they agreed that they would have an open relationship with as few restrictions as possible on the other's freedom to choose outside sexual partners.

For the first few years of their relationship, neither chose to interact with other partners. Then they met another couple who were similarly inclined and dated for over a year. When the other couple decided to close their marriage, Gina and Eric were grief stricken but happy that they still had each other. Although their marriage continues to be open in theory, they find that with each passing year they are less interested in including others. Eric says, "We have no rules against outside intimacy. It could happen again, but it would take someone very special to get our attention. The truth is, we're happy with what we've got and don't really feel a need for other sexual relationships."

Gina and Eric, according to my definition, are actually polyamorous even though the form their relationship has taken looks very much like a monogamous couple. To me, the most important aspect of polyamory is not how many partners a person has. Rather, it is the surrendering of conditioned beliefs about the form a loving relationship should take and allowing love itself to determine the form most appropriate for all parties. If the truth is that two people freely embrace sexual exclusivity not because somebody made them do it or because they're afraid of the consequences of doing something else, I would still consider that couple polyamorous.

The intention of polyamorous pioneers was not substituting one "should" for another. And yet that's exactly what many people are doing in communities where polyamory has become trendy. Instead of struggling to conform to a monogamous ideal and ideology, they find themselves struggling to conform to a nonmonogamous ideal and ideology. Meanwhile, young people who find polyamory either "too mainstream" or "too difficult" are rejecting the whole legacy and creating their own concepts, like *relationship anarchy* and *friends with benefits*, as we shall see in chapter 8. Labels, definitions, and organizations are useful insofar as they help us understand our experience and communicate about it, but what's the point of trading one rigid belief system for another?

Quite understandably, most people think that polyamory is about proclaiming their right to have more than one sexual partner or to have multipartner relationships. This might take the form of an open relationship where a couple, married or not, agrees to have additional lovers; a group marriage involving three or more people in one household; or an intimate network of couples and/or singles who have ongoing intimate relationships but don't live together. We'll look more closely at these variations later, but for now let's just say that polyamory implies an alternative to both serial monogamy and monogamy with secret affairs, which are the two most common relationship choices in the Western world.

To those of us who coined and popularized the term *polyamory*, the form the relationship takes is less important than the underlying values. The freedom of surrendering to love and allowing love—not just sexual passion, not just social norms and religious strictures, not just emotional reactions and unconscious conditioning—to determine the shape our intimate relationships take is the essence of polyamory. Polyamory is based on a decision to honor the many diverse ways loving relationships can evolve. Polyamory can take many forms, but as it was originally conceived, if deception or coercion is involved or if the people involved are out of integrity in any way, it's not polyamory no matter how many people are sexually involved with each other. These more subtle qualities have often gotten lost in the excitement and glamour of embracing sexual freedom, but they are crucial to understanding the deeper significance of polyamory.

A NEW PARADIGM FOR LOVE

The guilt and shame associated with premarital or extramarital sex and love is not quite a thing of the past, and neither is the lying and hiding that have accompanied these behaviors for centuries. Unfortunately, many old habits and patterns of relating have been translated into the polyamorous arena despite our idealistic vision for a future in which humans love each other unconditionally with passion and transparency and without possessiveness and control. Deep cultural change is a long-term affair. The increasing visibility of and acceptance for variations on the "one man, one woman, till death do us part" scenario has certainly decreased the shock value and threat that alternative choices once elicited, but we are still a long way from a true paradigm shift. In fact, few people believe that it's even possible for unconditional love and erotic love to coexist.

Those of us who are passionate about articulating a new paradigm for love and creating more tolerance for diversity in lovestyle choices agree that while monogamy is a wonderful option for some people some of the time, it's not the only valid possibility. The reality is that humans are not naturally monogamous. If we were, we would mate once, for life, and never for a moment consider doing anything else.

Polyamorous relationships, like monogamous ones, differ in their basic intentions and approaches. Some polyamorous relationships resemble traditional monogamous marriage in their emphasis on creating an impermeable boundary around the group, operating according to a well-defined set of rules (sometimes called a social contract), and expecting family members to replace individual desires with group agendas. I call this type of relationship "old paradigm" regardless of whether it is polyamorous or monogamous.

Other polyamorous relationships have a primary focus on using the relationships to further the psychological and spiritual development of the partners. These relationships tend to put more emphasis on responding authentically in the present moment, allowing for individual autonomy, and seeing loved ones as mirrors or reflections of oneself. These new paradigm relationships may also take either monogamous or polyamorous forms. Many people these days are in transition and find themselves attempting to blend elements of old and new paradigms as well as monogamous and polyamorous lovestyles, but these distinctions are useful in clarifying the direction in which we wish to move.

THE HUMAN ANIMAL AND ALL OUR RELATIONS

By the end of the twentieth century, scientific research on animal behavior and brain chemistry was providing strong confirmation of the troubling observation many of us had already made on our own—that lifelong monogamy is not natural for humans, nor is it for most other animals. Much publicity has been given to the sexual free-for-all enjoyed by our nearest genetic relatives: the bonobo chimpanzee. But nowhere in the animal kingdom do we find anything remotely resembling the phenomenon now called polyamory. Polyamory is a uniquely human phenomenon. Perhaps this is why conscious and consensual love-based intimate relating is generally left out of academic conversations on marriage and family.

For much of our evolutionary past, there were no centralized authorities dictating the terms of our sex lives. Rather, a variety of customs that supported local ecosystems gradually arose. In the last couple of millennia, organized religions, the medical establishment, and governments have increasingly taken charge of both sexual prohibitions and family structures. Nevertheless, in much of the world, men are still allowed to have more than one wife (called *polygyny* by anthropologists), and in a few places, women can have more than one husband (technically called *polyandry*). In countries where marriages are for couples only, both men and women often have secret extramarital affairs or divorce and marry another. All these patterns of mating and sexual activity can be found in the animal world. Some are more common than others, and while lifelong monogamy is rare, it does exist.

As David Barash and Judith Lipton discuss in their 2001 book *The Myth of Monogamy*, the advent of DNA testing to determine paternity was a major breakthrough in the study of animal mating patterns. Many species previously thought to be monogamous have since been found to be socially monogamous at best. That is, they may mate with a single individual, setting up housekeeping, coparenting, and sharing resources. But DNA testing along with more objective behavioral observation reveals that in many species both males and females have "secret affairs" often with other partnered individuals. Serial monogamy also occurs in the animal kingdom with both males and females "trading up" for a better mate when the opportunity arises.

Barash and Lipton's analysis of the proven absence of sexual exclusivity, even in most socially monogamous species, revolves around genetic programming. That is, both males and females will behave in ways that increase the likelihood of reproducing and the survival and successful mating of their offspring. Parenting and other social behavior as well as sexual habits are all strongly linked to genetic programming. Barash and Lipton also mention ecological considerations, what deep ecologists call the "carrying capacity of the land," as secondary influences on reproductive behaviors, and we'll return to this interesting factor in a later chapter.

The viewpoint that we could call DNA-driven sexual behavior is by no means new. But twentieth-century male sociobiologists frequently had blinders on when it came to the reproductive advantages accruing to females when mating with multiple males. It took women scientists[1] such as Dr. Sarah Hrdy, whose observations and interpretations often differed markedly from those made by men, to give us a more accurate picture. Hrdy was one of the first to note that among baboons, males would protect rather than attack the young of any female they had mated with. It's obvious to any unbiased observer that there are many genetic advantages in multiple matings for females as well as males.

Barash and Lipton, who are a male–female team, provide a more balanced perspective, putting to rest the outdated notion that females are naturally sexually exclusive. Instead, their data reveal that females, like males, are motivated to have more than one partner when doing so improves their access to resources and the quality of genetic material available to them.

Barash and Lipton also pose the fascinating question of why monogamy exists at all in any animals, including humans, and even go so far as to compare the reproductive advantages of monogamy, polygyny, and polyandry. Their new book, *Strange Bedfellows* (2009), focuses on the reproductive advantages of monogamy for humans. The animal behavior studies are illuminating. But while genetic programming dictates much more of our behavior than most of us like to admit, there are at least two serious limitations to animal research—and Barash and Lipton's analysis—for understanding human sexual behavior.

The first is that there are basically no known precedents either in the animal world or in so-called primitive cultures for mating or family groups that include more than one member of both genders, unless you consider the whole tribe as the group. For example, the concept of two males and two females bonding to reproduce and raise young is conspicuously absent from the literature. And while polyamory does not have to include multiple partners of both genders, it certainly can.

The reason for this, undoubtedly, is that while conflict between same-gender individuals competing to fertilize an egg, control territory, or obtain food and child care is generally present, when one male or female establishes dominance, he or she is able to assert him- or herself over the others more or less permanently, resulting in stable relationships where each individual knows how to behave.

But imagine what would happen if the alpha male or patriarch is not only ruling his harem but also constantly competing with another male whom he can't simply defeat and drive away but one with whom he needs to cooperate on an ongoing basis. A male who willingly submits to another becomes unattractive to females programmed to go for the male with the best genes. Similarly, an alpha female will generally not allow another female into her "home," and a nonalpha female will not succeed in preserving her freedom to have multiple mates in the face of inevitable resistance from males who want the genetic advantage of fertilizing all her eggs.

I've noticed these patterns in the cats I've lived with over the years. Recently, I adopted two female kittens whose mothers were sisters. They had been raised together since birth and were very bonded. Tillie is a very aggressive eater, gobbling her food as soon as it's placed in her dish and nosing her cousin out of the way. If it's something she especially likes, like fresh tuna, she makes growling noises while eating and guards the dish against intruders. Frances is quite content with this arrangement and patiently waits until her compatriot is finished eating to have whatever is left. They both love to sit with me and be petted. Tillie always sits on my shoulder or chest, while Frances takes the lower perch in my lap. When they play together, they wrestle and jump freely, but each knows her place when it comes to important resources, and there is never any conflict.

Years ago, I had two other cats who were sisters and got along well until they both had kittens. As soon as the kittens were weaned, Kali, the more dominant of the two, started attacking her sister many times a day until she drove her out of the house. Astarte finally found refuge with a neighbor, and Kali guarded her territory ferociously, refusing to submit to the male cats in the neighborhood except for Sand, our older male cat who lorded it over everyone.

Genetic programming is usually characterized as selfish. It's said that it's not interested in the good of the species, the happiness of others, or social justice but rather is ruled by Darwin's infamous survival-of-the-fittest dictum. Competition and the struggle for dominance, whether at the level of determining which sperm cells will fertilize an egg or which male has access to a particular female or whether the male or the female is calling the shots, has been the basis for most interpersonal interactions throughout our recorded history. Polyamory, on the other hand, involves a conscious decision to act altruistically, that is, to put the well-being of others on an equal par with one's own.

Another issue is that, increasingly, the association of human sexual behavior with reproduction is being broken. While most nonhuman sexual behavior still is linked with reproduction, a smaller and smaller percentage of human mating is intended to produce offspring. With longer life spans and better health, women are continuing to be sexually active long after fertility ceases. Greater independence for both genders means that enjoyment of sex, shared values and interests, and common avocations play a greater role than basic survival in sexual choices.

Meanwhile, many humans are deciding to have fewer children or no children at all, and when birth control pills and surgical solutions are used to control fertility and deodorants are used to control natural scents, our physiology is altered in such a way that genetic programming may be altered.

LOVE AND THE BRAIN

The effects of hormones and neurotransmitters have been increasingly well researched in the twenty-first century as the major mechanism by which genetic programming, as well as emotional reactions and environmental factors, exerts an effect on our sexual behavior. Hormones such as estrogen, testosterone, vasopressin, and dehydroepiandrosterone have long been known to influence our sexual desires and habits. Oxytocin is strongly linked to bonding. Neurotransmitters such as dopamine, norepinephrine, and phenylethylamine have been identified as mediators for infatuation or romantic love. Tiny molecules called pheromones, which enter our bodies through the nose, independently of our conscious awareness of odors, also influence our sexual attractions and choices.

The question is no longer whether sex hormones affect our behavior but rather to what extent we have any conscious choice about our sexual decisions at all. For example, high testosterone levels may incline some people to seek out multiple partners, while vasopressin may influence others to bond with only one. No doubt the degrees of freedom vary from person to person and involve relationships between hormone levels, consciousness levels, and environmental factors. The very extensive conversations on "free will" in spiritual, psychological, and philosophical venues are beyond the scope of this book. Suffice it to say that many of our most respected and influential spiritual leaders say that free will is an illusion and that we only imagine we are making choices after the behavior has already occurred.[2]

Scientific data strongly suggest that, as sex therapist and researcher Dr. Theresa Crenshaw puts it, "when you fall in love or in lust it isn't merely an emotional event. Your various hormones, each with unique features to contribute, get in bed with you too."[3] Dr. Helen Fisher divides love into three categories that correspond to different hormones and brain systems. Her analysis of the data suggests that high androgen and estrogen levels generate lust, romantic love correlates with high dopamine and norepinephrine and low serotonin, and attachment is driven by oxytocin and vasopressin. To make matters more complicated, these three systems interact. For example, testosterone can "kickstart the two love neurotransmitters while an orgasm can elevate the attachment hormone," according to Fisher. "Don't copulate with people you don't want to fall in love with," she warns.[4]

Scientists also tell us that the intensity of romantic love that many couples experience early on, which is fueled by endorphins, naturally diminishes after a couple of years. Oxytocin levels then support a few more years of attachment, rising with the birth of each new child, perhaps accounting for worldwide peaks in divorce rates after four and seven years of marriage as bonding between partners loses some of its biochemical boost. If affectionate touch, sexual activity, and orgasms also decline over time, oxytocin levels will further decline.

Vasopressin, which has been called "the monogamy molecule" because it's been identified as the cause of lifelong mating patterns in male prairie voles, has also been implicated in human bonding. Swedish researcher Hasse Walum[5] reports that in a study of 552 pairs of male twins, those with a gene reducing the effect of vasopressin scored lower on a psychological test measuring bonding. The women they were married to also reported lower levels of marital quality. As a result, there has been speculation that vasopressin levels may play in a role in determining whether a man is monogamous.

Marnia Robinson, author of *Peace between the Sheets*, advocates that both men and women withhold orgasm during sexual exchanges to short-circuit the brain circuitry, leading to a decline of interest in a partner once they've habituated to each other. She theorizes that the human brain, unlike the bonobo brain, is wired for pair bonding with a specific type of dopamine receptor that creates addictive-like cravings for one's mate. But as with any physical addiction, the "fix" loses its potency over time. Robinson speculates that by withholding dopamine-releasing orgasms while increasing oxytocin-releasing touch and affection, bonding can prevail over the "craving" for new and different sexual stimulation.[6] If Robinson's hypothesis is correct, it goes a long way toward explaining why women, who are generally less likely than men to reach orgasm through intercourse or to reach orgasm at all if their lover is unskilled, are reputed to be more likely to remain attached, while their male partners seek variety.

While love, sex, and relationships are clearly influenced by many factors in addition to genetic variations, hormones and neurotransmitters, and pharmaceutical and recreational drugs, most experts agree that we would be foolish to ignore the role of biochemistry.

IS INFIDELITY MONOGAMY?

Is infidelity monogamy? What about serial monogamy? These may sound like silly questions, but with as many as 70 percent of all couples experiencing extramarital affairs, monogamy has been redefined. Most of these couples consider themselves to be monogamous, as do couples who divorce and remarry others. Clearly, their behavior does not match their identities. As long our society stigmatizes people—and especially women—who tell the truth about their nonmonogamous desires and activities, it's likely that people will choose more acceptable labels even if they are misleading to say the least.

According to the 1999 U.S. Census, almost half of all marriages are remarriages for at least one of the spouses. While divorce rates are higher in the United States than in most other countries, serial monogamy is a worldwide trend. And one of the leading causes of divorce is infidelity. The original meaning of monogamy was to mate and be sexually exclusive for life. Divorcing and remarrying was originally called serial polygamy, not serial monogamy.

We could argue whether all marriages should continue for a lifetime, but that's not the issue I want to raise here. Rather, I am pointing to the false connection many people make between monogamy and fidelity.

Monogamy and commitment are often considered synonymous as well. To me, faithfulness has more to do with honesty, respect, and loyalty than sexual exclusivity, and commitment is about keeping agreements. The content of the agreement is irrelevant as far as commitment is concerned. Somehow, we've really gotten confused when relationships that include secret extramarital affairs are considered monogamous and those that end in divorce are considered committed monogamous marriages.

Of course, people who identify as monogamous have no corner on infidelity. Those who attempt to practice polyamory can also find themselves having secret affairs, which is all the more disheartening to partners who imagined that their couple relationship was based on honesty and consensual extramarital relating. Ellen and her husband Doug had been happily married for twelve years, and while they'd agreed from the beginning that their marriage would be open, neither had gone beyond the playful flirtation stage.

Suddenly, unexpectedly Ellen found herself head over heels in love with William, a man whom both had been acquainted with for years. She'd kept the depth of her feelings a secret from Doug for several months, not wanting to upset him and afraid that he would interfere with her newfound joy. Meanwhile, William, knowing that they had an open marriage, assumed that Doug was fully informed. When Ellen finally confessed that she was in love with William, Doug predictably felt angry and betrayed, feared that she would leave him, and wanted to retreat to monogamy. The habit of keeping secrets can be deeply engrained, even when couples agree to have an open relationship.

SWINGING

For many people, *polyamory* is just another word for *swinging*. In fact, prior to the invention of the word *polyamory* in the early 1990s, the word *swinging*, when it came into use in the 1970s, did mean much the same thing *polyamory* now implies. Like polyamory, the definition of swinging and swingers has evolved through the portrayal of these lifestyles in the popular media.

I know this because shortly after the publication of my book *Love without Limits* in 1992, I gave a talk at the annual Lifestyles Conference to promote it. In my talk, I discussed my impression that while swinging shares the values of honesty and consensual decision making with polyamory, it differs from polyamory in two ways. First, swingers generally had sex first and perhaps became friends later, whereas polyamorists became friends first and maybe had sex afterward. Second, swinging, while allowing for sexual non-monogamy, demanded emotional monogamy. That is, in swinging, falling in love with a partner other than your spouse is forbidden. In polyamory, the word itself suggests that loving all of your partners is appropriate.

While my description is certainly true for some swingers, when my talk concluded, I was surrounded by polite but angry swingers, including many leaders in the swing movement who informed me that their way of practicing swinging had always been identical to what I was now calling polyamory. In fact, some of them were involved in intimate networks that were almost as old as I was at the time. The media, they said, were responsible for sensationalizing the lifestyle and presenting it as shallow and coldhearted.

The same could now be said of polyamory, but in all fairness, I have to admit that some people who have adopted the polyamory label have sex instead of developing lasting friendships and don't always treat their partners in a loving way. And there are many people who call themselves swingers but who have committed relationships with a circle of people beyond their primary partner. In addition, I know of many people who have ongoing sexualoving relationships with several people and also have a series of casual sexual encounters with new people. Others troll for prospects for polyamorous relationships by attending swing conventions that are generally held at more upscale locations, more entertaining, less introspective, and better attended than polyamory conferences.

Another difference between polyamory and swinging is that at least in present-day swinging, it's all about couples. In order to attend most swinging events, you have to be a male/female pair. Honestly, I'm not sure to what extent the "couples-only" policy is an effective way of discouraging single men from swarming to these events and to what extent it is a strategy for managing jealousy by eliminating, at least in theory, participants who may be seeking a new mate. Polyamorous gatherings, because they are less sexually oriented, are less attractive to people who are primarily seeking sex. Additionally, in polyamory there is usually a conscious choice not to support the culturally pervasive emphasis on coupling up.

Clearly, there is no sharp divide between polyamory and swinging, with some people practicing or identifying with both lifestyles and others choosing labels according to their circumstances or their history or for no apparent reason at all. The distinction may be helpful to some, but it's not something you can rely on to be meaningful.

Nora and Jim's story is a case in point. Nora recalls, "When the kids went off to college we realized we'd bankrupted our marriage. That's a dangerous time for marriages breaking up, and Jim and I decided we needed to spend more time together and focus on each other after all these years of being in the polyamorous community and having other lovers. We'd drifted apart. His needs were being met by Andrea, his girlfriend of seven years, but my other partners weren't working out for me, and I stopped seeing them."

At that time, Nora told Jim, "If you'd rather be with her, there's the door. I only want you to be here if you want to be." They spent a year in counseling together, and Nora invited Andrea to join them, but Andrea declined and "wrote herself out of the script." Nora says she hadn't planned to exclude Andrea but did want to reclaim her connection with her husband and feels badly about how that relationship ended.

"I've always been kind of a tribal person," Nora explains. "I still have a circle of close friends from childhood. I liked the idea of having more friends around who we could also have sex with, but it really hadn't worked out for me. Jim's and my sex life had always been good, there was nothing lacking in our relationship, we just started wondering what more there could be to life. At first it felt very inclusive, very spontaneous, we were doing it together with the first couple we dated. And I was always 'open' with my other lovers, but Jim was in a closed relationship with Andrea, who didn't want him to see other women besides me.

"After we got our marriage back on track five years ago, Jim wanted to try swinging, which was something we'd never done and which he couldn't do with Andrea. I wasn't really interested, but I was a good sport, so I went along with it. I didn't like it much, but after a couple months we met a couple at a swing club who we now see every weekend. It's turned out to be the way I always imagined polyamory could be but never was. No stress, no strain, no drama. There's a lot of trust and comfort. We have a great time with them, and there's a lot of love and support. The first year it was mostly just great sex. They'd been swinging for a long time and were a very happy, stable couple. Polyamory just wasn't on their map. They'd never heard of it. I was cautious after my previous experiences and wanted to go very slowly. I think they were open to more with us before we were. In the second year we expanded to dinners, sleepovers, meeting each other's kids, and taking vacations together. They've become our best friends, we're in love with each other, we're bonded. Our kids love them, and their kids like us too. Their nineteen-year-old daughter recently asked them matter-of-factly if they were swingers and if they had sex with us. When they said yes and yes, she simply nodded and said, 'Cool.'"

THE ECOLOGY OF INTIMATE RELATIONSHIPS

While twenty-first-century mainstream Judeo-Christian doctrines concur in prescribing monogamy as the only appropriate form for marriage, this was not always the case. Insisting that everyone be monogamous is analogous to monocropping in agriculture where large corporate farms plant thousands of acres with just one crop, destroying the complex interrelated diversity of species that have coevolved healthy, sustainable ecosystems over many generations.

These are some of the forms intimate relationships often take when people allow themselves to find a niche appropriate for the unique individuals involved. Note that some of these forms may interact. For example, a couple in an open marriage may also be part of an intimate network.

Open Marriage or Open Relationship

Both of these are nonexclusive couple relationships, the main difference being whether the couple is married. In this scenario, the partners have agreed that each can have outside partners. A wide variety of ground rules and restrictions may apply.

Gina and Eric, whom we met earlier in this chapter, have an open marriage. Even though they don't currently have outside sexual partners, they have a clear agreement that allows for this possibility. Mark and Nancy also have an open marriage, but in contrast to Gina and Eric, who discuss each situation as it arises, Mark and Nancy have a list of guidelines each is committed to follow. Their basic rule is that they ask the other's permission before making a date with someone else. Each has the option to meet a potential new partner before giving permission. At times, they have had "standing" dates on a certain night of the week with a long-term lover, but Mark and Nancy always have the option to veto the date night if they feel a need for more time with each other. They have also agreed to always be home by midnight.

Intimate Network

This is a lovestyle in which several ongoing relationships coexist but usually people do not live together, or they may share housing or land as roommates or community mates rather than as partners. Sometimes all members of the informal group eventually become lovers. Sometimes individuals have only one or a few sexualoving partners within the group, but they generally have close friendships. The group can include singles, couples, moresomes, or a mixture. Another way to describe an intimate network would be as a circle of sexualoving friends. The intimate network is similar to what futurist F. M. Esfandiary called a *mobilia* in the 1970s and what young Swedish activist Andie Nordgren calls *relationship anarchy* in the twenty-first-century.

Bruce, Jane, Cindy, Rebecca, Richard, and Harry have been friends and lovers for over twelve years. Cindy was introduced to Bruce and Jane by her ex-husband Jim, who has also been part of this intimate network at times. Bruce and Jane are a committed couple in an open relationship, and both were lovers of Cindy's for several years, although this relationship has become a mostly nonsexual close friendship since Cindy got together with Harry six years ago. Rebecca is an old friend of Jane's who became sexually involved with Bruce two years ago, and Richard is a single man who is lovers with Jane and Cindy and occasionally Harry.

Group Marriage

A group marriage is a committed, long-term, primary relationship that includes three or more adults of any gender in a marriage-like relationship. A group marriage can be open or closed to outside sexual partners. It may revolve around one central person who is primary with all the others (called a "V"), or each person may be equally close to every other person involved.

Peter and Candy had been married for twenty-three years and raised two children when Peter fell in love with Jessica, who was ten years his junior. He knew immediately that he wanted to include Jessica into his already happy marriage with Candy rather than divorcing Candy to be with

Jessica. Both women were skeptical but willing to explore developing a relationship of their own. It turned out that Candy and Jessica quickly became best friends, are very compatible, and love spending time together. They experimented sexually, both alone and with Peter, but have concluded that they are more interested in Peter sexually than in each other. They do enjoy sharing Peter in bed, which is just fine with Peter. Jessica moved into Peter and Candy's large home four years ago and has decided to go back to school and get a law degree so that she can join Peter and Candy's legal practice. The three have agreed to have an open marriage, but so far they are too busy enjoying each other to have any interest in seeking new partners.

Triad

Three sexualoving partners who may be in any combination of primary, secondary, or nonhierarchical relationships. A triad may be open or closed, but if it's a polyamorous triad, it's more ongoing than a one-night ménage à trois. It can be strictly heterosexual or homosexual, or it can be the choice of two same-gender bisexuals and an opposite-gender heterosexual.

Peter, Candy, and Jessica are an example of a triad as well as a group marriage, and so are John, Eli, and Carol, who are all singles who share a flat in Helsinki. John and Carol met in college six years ago and became friends and lovers. When Carol went away to graduate school, they separated, and John decided to explore an intimate relationship with Eli. When Carol returned to Helsinki and met Eli, they were immediately attracted and decided to experiment with a three-way relationship that included John. After two years, they decided to try living together and are now considering having a child together.

2

WHO CHOOSES POLYAMORY, AND WHY?

The diversity that characterizes the universe of those who've adopted polyamorous styles of relating reveals itself most clearly when we address the wide variety of motivations people may have for choosing polyamory. Some may harbor hopes that polyamory will allow them to avoid dealing with problematic personal issues or that it will solve problems in an existing relationship, but this is rarely the case. In a few cases, however, polyamory does allow people to create healthy and functional relationships they probably could not have managed otherwise. In others, one partner reluctantly agrees to polyamory to win the affections of the other, secretly hoping that this unwelcome twist will magically vanish once they are committed to each other. Some are consciously or unconsciously creating a situation in which they can heal childhood wounds or replicate the large extended family they grew up in.

Some want a stable and nurturing environment in which to raise their children. Some use polyamory to mask or excuse addictions to sex, work, or drama, while others seek utopian or spiritual rewards or want to take a stand for cultural change. Others are simply doing what's fun and what comes naturally for them or are rebelling against religious prohibitions or family expectations. Some use polyamory as a weapon in a power struggle or to punish a controlling partner. Some want to keep their erotic life alive and vital while in long-term committed relationships or to fulfill sexual or

emotional desires they can't meet with only one person or with their existing partner. Some are trying to make up for developmental gaps or to balance unequal sex drives. Some people do not start out consciously choosing
polyamory at all but find that polyamory has chosen them.

As I was sitting down to write this chapter, I received an e-mail from a
woman who had recently read some of the articles about polyamory that
are posted on my website. Her comments seem the perfect place to begin
this discussion on why people choose polyamory. This woman, who I'll call
Kate, was grateful to find a confirmation of her own experience of polyamory as a spiritual path. "I don't think I've ever engaged in anything that
has prompted more self-reflection and intense personal growth than has
polyamory," she concludes.

The blessing and the curse of polyamory is that love that includes more
than one tends to illuminate those dark shadows that many would prefer
to ignore. While some people deliberately seek out polyamorous relationships for the purpose of freeing themselves and their children from the
neuroses arising from typical nuclear family dynamics, most inadvertently
discover that polyamory provides a very fertile environment for replicating
any dysfunctional patterns carried over from the parental triangle experienced in their family of origin.

Men may find childhood competition with Dad for the attention of
Mom rekindled when they relate with a woman who has another lover. If
they unconsciously begin to act out the old childhood script of competition
with the man for the heart of the woman, an unpleasant and painful drama
is likely to unfold. If instead they can consciously find ways to support each
other in basking in the richness of loving both each other (which need
not include sexuality) and the woman and to creatively manage the only
truly limited resource—that is, *time*, not love—a more enjoyable outcome
is possible. Many men have strong competitive instincts that they have
been socialized to express very directly. Women frequently have the same
strong competitive urge, but women's socialization has driven competition
underground, and it often comes out sideways, making it even more challenging to overcome. Unresolved sibling rivalries can also be rekindled in
polyamorous relating. These are situations in which an ounce of prevention
is worth a pound of cure, so it behooves people who are contemplating
polyamory to heal their family of origin issues first.

Abundant love can bring out our shadow in ways that have little to do
with jealousy and competition. I once spent a week vacationing with a man

whom I was newly in love with and another couple who both of us were attracted to and who I'd been very close to for several years. I eagerly anticipated our time together, imagining how wonderful it would be to enjoy the company of three people I loved and who loved me. After a few days, I found myself feeling more and more uncomfortable. Feelings of unworthiness I never knew I had began overwhelming me. My usual calm and self-confident self had disappeared, and in its place was an anxious and insecure stranger. At first, I didn't understand what was happening and tried to push these troubling feelings away, but they only got stronger. I found myself wondering whether I deserved this much love. Was I really good enough for him and him and her? Finally, I tearfully confessed that my self-esteem had hit an all-time low. Held in three pairs of loving arms, I took the invitation to dive into my shadow and experienced firsthand the legendary power of love to light up the dark corners of the psyche, shedding healing light on that which has been hidden.

SELF-ACTUALIZING POLYAMORISTS

Nancy and Darrell are a good example of a couple who deliberately chose polyamory for its opportunities for growth as well as to allow a broader sexual context within their marriage. Both were virgins in their early twenties when they married forty years ago. After ten years of being happily monogamous, while attending a relationship seminar they discovered that neither one was invested in sexual exclusivity. It turned out that they had simply defaulted to monogamy, as do so many people, and once they took a look at it, they realized that their only reason for continuing to be monogamous was fear of the unknown. Confident of their love, their compatibility, their communication skills, and their commitment to each other, they decided to open their marriage. It's less common now than in the past for couples to have no sexual experience before marrying, but I know of many such couples who have found in polyamory a way to jointly embark on the adventures they missed out on in their youth.

Nancy reports, "When Darrell told me he wanted to know what it would be like to make love to a red-headed woman, I responded, 'So do I, but she doesn't have to be a redhead.' I had squelched my bisexual being to satisfy the demands of monogamy. It was time for both of us to explore!" They began by checking out swinging. Nancy continues, "Swinging was easily accessible. We were uncomfortable with the idea of having sex with strangers, so we chose off-premise clubs, which meant we got to dance, flirt, chat, and get acquainted with potential partners. We both preferred to become friends before making love. The owner of our chosen club explained at the start of each dance, 'When you want to cum, you need to go.' That was fine with us!

"I also ran an ad in an underground paper and met a woman with whom I hoped to discover that elusive chemistry so we could become lovers. Instead, she became my best friend as she and Darrell became lovers, and we established a polyamorous trio. We experienced a sequence of three trios, two of which lasted many years." Nancy is careful to let me know that they're still friends with one of these women after twenty-four years, although she is now in a monogamous marriage. Another has been part of their lives for twelve years, although it's been eight years since they've been lovers. Nancy and Darrell also have relationships with several couples that have gone on for anywhere from two to twenty years, so she's had many opportunities to explore making love with women.

While Nancy and Darrell consciously chose polyamory as an opportunity to grow together and to deepen their own bond while exploring committed sexualoving relationships with others, they didn't immediately realize that polyamory would become a spiritual practice. When I first met them about fifteen years ago, they were seeking help in releasing and transforming jealousy. Nancy appeared the more emotional of the two, but both exuded a sensible, good-humored sincerity. Through cultivating compersion (a term describing an emotion that is the opposite of jealousy and discussed further in chapter 6) and incorporating the concept of "honoring the Divine in each other and in every one of our partners," polyamory became a doorway into spiritual growth for Nancy and Darrell, leading Nancy to write an article, "Spiritual Partnership," for *Loving More* magazine, in which she writes, "Within Spiritual Partnership, mutual spiritual growth takes precedence over comfort and security and total honesty becomes part of the bond. Spiritual partners are committed to a personal growth dynamic, even if it is not 'comfortable and secure.' Within this paradigm, monogamy becomes a choice instead of a mandate and nontraditional relationships naturally evolve through partners becoming committed to honestly sharing at a heart level."[1]

Nancy continues, "Our relationship has been open for about thirty years now, and we are still deeply committed to each other and to our extended family. Sometimes that commitment means listening lovingly to someone who has lost his job; it may mean my accepting that Darrell will spend time loving a woman who has decided she no longer wants to spend much time with me. Although her decision may have bruised my ego, becoming peaceful despite that bruise is part of my own personal growth process. If poly is a spiritual path, my ego is less involved when personal and spiritual growth remain paramount. This makes it easier to let go of jealousy and allow compersion to counter fear, which results in less drama.

"We're now in our sixties and retired, which allows us to have a lot of time and energy for extended relationships. Ironically, during the summer, I am pretty much monogamous by choice as Darrell continues his relationship with two women. One of those two is a heart-centered friend of mine; the other prefers to have her connection limited to Darrell. In the other seasons, we share loving energy with several other couples and an occasional single."

Nancy is a retired therapist, so she and Darrell sometimes act as coaches for couples who want to explore how to have an open, loving relationship with each other (and include others) with minimum drama. She feels that "one extremely important part of practicing successful polyamory is the recognition that change is the only constant in multiple relationships. Inherent in each polyamorous beginning is an unplanned ending. As we age, lovers die, become geographically challenged through moving away, or decide to become monogamous, which means we shift into a nonsexual friendship or lose the relationship." Nancy and Darrell also value their spiritual partnerships with polyamorous friends who have never been lovers but where the love is deep and complete nevertheless.

Kamala and Michael are a happy and successful thirty-something-year-old couple with a three-year-old son. They've been in an open marriage for seven years and have a large extended family of friends and lovers. Kamala is also a relationship coach and poly activist who has made many media appearances in recent years. She is following the trail I blazed a decade earlier, braving the slings and arrows of those who believe strongly in monogamy as a religious ideal. She's been accused of trying to convert others to nonmonogamy, trying to prove something to the religious right, and taking advantage of the free publicity to market her books and DVDs. Kamala retorts, "I have no idea what difference it will make in the long run. What I know is that I love my life. My husband, my

son, and most of my lovers are truly happy." Kamala says she's motivated
by a strong desire to be a "voice for freedom and love in the world. I'm
willing to be misunderstood, misquoted or misrepresented, whatever it
takes. . . . I'm willing to show up and be seen" if it makes the world a
better place.[2]

Sonia Song grew up in Communist China. She was raised to be a good
party member but lost faith in the Cultural Revolution after the horrors
of the Tiananmen Square massacre. Eventually, she found her way to
California, where she first sought me out about ten years ago because she
was looking for an ethical way to expand beyond a loveless and sexless
marriage with a husband who didn't want to divorce for practical reasons.
Sonia has long since extricated herself from that marriage and found
more compatible partners but continues to choose polyamory because
it feels right to her. We'll hear more about Sonia's polyamorous life in a
later chapter, but for now the conclusion from her book, *Donkey Baby*,
is an eloquent expression of the idealism that inspires some people to
choose polyamory.

"In the Orient the butterfly is a symbol of love and sex. In the West it's
a symbol of transformation. I feel like a butterfly in both senses. My life
journey began being carried in a basket on a donkey's back in China during
my parents' march to Beijing with the People's Liberation Army. Today I
am actively involved in the global peace, justice, and environmental movement in California. Have I found love? I think love has found me. And I
have gained a greater appreciation of the human spirit that carries each of
us in search for our own path. For me, the polyamorous way of relating
to people is my utopian dream come true, a revolutionary approach in human relations, as well as a powerful political statement: If we love and feel
loved, we will be peaceful; furthermore, if we can bring that spirit of love
and peace to formulating and implementing social, economic, and political
policies, positive changes will follow. Today I'm living my values by enjoying a joyful polyamorous lifestyle, politically active, ecologically conscious,
and spiritually grounded."[3]

C. T. Butler, who is now in his fifties, has lived polyamorously and been
actively engaged in working for social change for his entire adult life. In
1981, he cofounded the Food Not Bombs collective, which is still going
strong around the world as a grassroots organization to provide free veg-
etarian meals for the hungry and raise awareness about homelessness as
well as protesting war and military spending.

C.T. reports that for two years in the early days of Food Not Bombs, the collective was run by three men and three women who shared a large house and whose relationships included sexual involvement with each other in one way or another. They went so far in challenging the status quo that they had the experiment of not having their own personal bedrooms in the house. C.T. recalls, "Downstairs, we had the kitchen, dining room, living room, and study; upstairs, we had the sleeping room, the sex room, the library/meditation room, and the music room. We all slept together in one big bed in the sleeping room, and sometimes, some would sleep in the sex room or music room. There were others moving in or moving out of the collective all the time."

While many of the young people who formed the Food Not Bombs collective were already lovers, they were "seasoned activists" who viewed their sexually radical lifestyle as a precaution against infiltration. C.T. recalls that "we were quite concerned about infiltration at the time and felt that the willingness to be sexual and deeply intimate with everyone else in the collective was a way to prevent infiltration. Obviously, we did not think it was absolutely foolproof; we just thought it was helpful. However, that does not mean we required everyone to have sex with everyone else in the collective; it was that we were interested in experimenting with sexual relations in an outside-the-box way, and we saw the usefulness of this experimenting in strengthening our bonds and our effectiveness as political activists. Therefore, in practice, if someone was unwilling to experiment, they were not suitable collective members. If they were comfortable with open relationships and had a willingness to experiment sexually, as demonstrated by their behavior, then we assumed they were very unlikely to be an agent of the state."

In keeping with their anarchist politics, the collective were strong adherents of consensus decision making. Any member could call a meeting called a group-group, where everyone would engage in a discussion that could not end until everyone agreed on a resolution, which might mean two or three days with breaks only for eating and sleeping. C.T. reports that these group-groups were called only maybe five times in two years to address things like "dealing with a sexual predator, kicking a member out, and sexism."[4]

C.T. says that jealousy was never much of a problem for him because of his "political analysis of life." He explains that, "from early adulthood, I realized that possessive behaviors and the idea that one person could control the behavior of another because of the concept of marriage was really just another form of slavery, one person owning another. I have never wanted to control or have another person all for myself. With regard to the jealousy my partners would feel, I was very patient and clear that jealousy is primarily based on fear. I would take the time to help my partner uncover her fear and manage it so that it would either go away or, at least, not destroy our relationship. Generally, that worked pretty well." During the 1980s and 1990s, he helped start polyamory discussion groups throughout New England, lived in a series of polyamorous families, and fathered several children. For C.T., polyamory was as much a tool for political activism as a means of personal gratification.

POLYAMORY AND SEX ADDICTION

Not all polyamorists claim to be as well prepared or idealistic in their motivations as Nancy and Darrell or Kamala and Michael, Sonia Song, or C. T. Butler. In some cases, polyamory becomes a context for the unconscious playing out of the classic addict and codependent drama; in others, the dynamics show a mixture of conflicting motivations to satisfy an addiction alongside more altruistic, growth-oriented, or utopian agendas.

Thelma first sought my advice on informational resources about polyamory because a year or so into their relationship, her boyfriend had come out to her as polyamorous, and she wanted to learn more about it. "I am *not* polyamorous," she told me. "I have enough difficulty with one relationship at a time, and I would go completely unconscious in a number of simultaneous relationships. But I'm in love with him, and he wants polyamory, so I'm trying to be open minded about it." I suggested a few books and websites, offered to put her on my mailing list, and suggested she let me know if she wanted some coaching in navigating this unfamiliar territory. About two years later, Thelma sought help from a therapist.

Several years after that, Thelma looked me up again, asking what I thought about sex addiction. I responded that I was very disturbed by the presence of sex addiction in the polyamory community, saying that while most polyamorous people are *not* addicts, it was a significant problem and one that often came up for discussion in my workshops. Although I wish sex addiction was never an issue in polyamory, the truth is that polyamory does provide a convenient cover story for addicts who are generally in denial about having an addiction. It's easy to justify sexual obsession by calling it polyamory. A handful of sex addicts can wreak havoc in a community, especially when people are still operating out of conditioning that forbids the sharing of "family secrets" out of misguided respect for confidentiality. Polyamory offers a venue in which sex addicts can begin at least to tell the truth about what they're doing instead of carrying on secret affairs. I prefer to put a positive spin on it by seeing that bringing their destructive, addictive behavior out into the open is the first step toward healing, but unfortunately it can get messy and hurtful for those who are hoping for love and instead find callousness.

After hearing my opinions, Thelma decided she'd like to tell me about her own experience. "I can well describe what it is like, how it feels to be the substance that a sex addict uses to engage in his addiction. If I could curtail even one person's suffering by doing so, it would be worth revisiting the whole ugly mess which I finally put behind me two years ago," she told me. For Thelma, the idea that she was attempting a polyamorous relationship that would involve a potentially painful confrontation with her own jealousy but would be well worth it in the end allowed her to be drawn into an abusive relationship. A man with more empathy and integrity would have either told her about his sexual activity with other women before she became so deeply involved or curtailed his sexual adventures until he had disengaged with her once it became apparent she was suffering so intensely. Here is her story in her own words.

"This is about loving a man who was and is a sex addict. It is a story that ends with loving myself for the first time ever. Into the wounded and forgotten places, into the hated cesspools that I had tried to paper over and pretend out of existence. Of course, I cannot know if there was another way I could have gotten where I am. I certainly wish that it had not been so painful, so depraved. I will never know what might have been had I not had this set of experiences.

"The relationship began with more hope than I had ever dared. Looking back, I can see now how frightened I really was. In hindsight, I can see scores of warning signs that I ignored, misinterpreted, reimagined to fit my high hopes that covered my desperation for enduring love. The external events and my reactions changed over the six years with this man. At first I reacted quickly; I was indignant, angry, fully expecting him to change his behavior. Surely I could show him these errors, and he would correct them. Right?

"I later changed to defensive behaviors. This is the longest chapter of all—this is the place that I lost myself utterly trying to maintain a relationship that was much more in my head than in my life. Every day was so full of hurt and despair and calculated prevention that there was precious little of myself left in everyday life. Finally, I devolved to a conviction that this misery, this unremitting effort with horrific results, was going to be my entire life. He would never hear my agony, see the effects he was having upon me. If he could just know how much I was hurting, surely he would stop, I still hoped weakly. No one could be so cruel, could they? Surely my efforts would matter; this would all have a satisfactory ever-after ending, happy and glowing.

"For years, his compulsive flirtations, the online pornography, the obsessive masturbation in the shower, the dates with other women when he was out of town, the secretive seductions and ongoing attempts to have other lovers, sometimes successful, the "friendships" with coworkers and business associates kept me off balance. I worked with every ounce of ability I possessed (or could borrow from others) to contain this behavior. I was so desperate for help maintaining my relationship, I compromised my friendships, my values, my integrity and ultimately any shreds of respect for myself.

"Then, finally, he upped the ante. He announced he was going to spend the night with a 'Tantra' practitioner who was clearly besotted with him. She sold her sexual services for money and called it Tantra. He had enticed her overtures, and she was one of those women who had a sad need to involve herself with unavailable men. She knew that we were living together and executed this rendezvous anyway. He was enthralled with her flattery, so much so that he responded to my pleas to not hurt me so deeply with threats of violence instead of empathy for the pain I was displaying. He had been violent in the not-too-distant past, so inward again went the humiliation, the pain. There was no more room, I could not hold another ounce of pain. In utter despair, with no way to stop the pain, I planned to commit suicide that night rather than have to be tortured one more minute. I had invested everything that I had into this relationship, and he was throwing me away and everything that I had worked diligently for six years for a night with a prostitute.

"So how did this begin? How did I come to this place? How did I go from having an admittedly interesting life to the precipice of suicide? What about all the in-between things that happened? There are places that I can explain with great fervor, and even a dash of humor, some sweeping geographies that can be described with grand dispassion, corners that remain shrouded to me still, and places that I will never ever, ever have the vantage place to see. There are places that are for others to define and shine light upon. There were places, dark and cavernous, that I fumbled through and emerged in spite of my lack of navigation skills or even the ability to see fifteen seconds into the future. I call those places grace. There are places that I revisited ad nauseam, ad infinitum, failing an astounding number of times to avoid because I was trying yet *another* fix/cure/technique/ploy to prevent the recurring addictive scenarios."

Thelma's story is the polar opposite of Nancy and Darrell's, chock full of drama, manipulation, and misery. In addition to being a story about addiction, it's a story about a woman who knows very clearly that she wants monogamy but is so desperate for love that she tries to tolerate an inconsiderate, nonmonogamous partner, hoping she can somehow change him. Chances are she would not have gotten involved had she known he was unwilling to be monogamous, but by the time she found out, she was hooked. Some individuals struggling with sex addiction behave more responsibly but still find healthy polyamorous relationships impossible.

Alex is a handsome, charismatic man in his late forties who is a professional entertainer. His outgoing personality, sexy voice, and boyish charm make him a magnet for women. When he first heard about polyamory ten years ago, he was newly single and fascinated. But after almost losing his new partner, Dawn, he decided he'd better take another look at his motivations for choosing polyamory. Dawn, like Thelma, tried valiantly to accept Alex's desire for polyamory, but she heeded the red flags and the coaching I gave her to insist that Alex get his addictive behavior under control before agreeing to continue having an open relationship.

Alex recalls that "I immediately resonated with the concept of open, free sexual relationships that could foster deeper communication and intimacy. I felt so at home in the poly community, and for the first time, I didn't feel shame about desiring to love more than one. What I didn't realize at the time was that I had a huge need for the romantic intrigue associated with new relationships. It wasn't so much the sex, although that part was great, but the high of being newly in love that just took me over. I was able to hide behind polyamory when what I was mostly looking for was escape from feeling I wasn't enough. Once I started paying closer attention to what was going on inside me, I found out that as soon as I'd start feeling bad about myself, I'd drown my low self-esteem in a new infatuation.

"For me, the idea of polyamory makes sense and feels right since I'd rather face my jealousy than force my partner to be monogamous. Plus, I like the idea of sharing my love and sexuality with more than one lover. I have a lot to give, and giving it just feels good. Dawn feels the same way about sharing love but not about facing her jealousy. For her, sharing love is a choice, but for me there seems to more of an uncontrollable drive for the excitement and emotional and sexual juice. I realized that for me it was not a simple choice only after destroying over a dozen beautiful love relationships, a business partnership, and a teen ministry largely because of my 'need' for poly freedom.

"When Dawn and I got together in 2000, we began to explore healthier, more conscious ways for me to get my poly desires met and not be addictive, inconsiderate, and compulsive. After over six years of emotional roller coasting, we both finally realized that I was not able to do poly in a healthy way since my addictive behaviors and emotional wounds always seemed to prevail. At that point, after an ultimatum from Dawn, I chose sobriety from poly life. Since then, the dramas have all but ceased along with all the shame that was associated with feeling out of control and hurting others. In addition, my relationship with Dawn has deepened and recently gotten even more sexual and passionate. I do crave new sexual experiences from time to time, and all I have to do is think of the pain, chaos, and drama, and I'm back to happy sobriety."

For Alex, polyamory did provide a context in which he was able to see that it was not so much the jealousy and possessiveness of his partner who was willing to selectively and responsibly include others into their intimacy, nor was it the judgments of society, which were essentially reversed in the polyamory community, that stood between him and his sexual freedom. Rather, he became aware for the first time that nonmonogamy was workable only if he could heal the childhood wounds that led him to compulsively lose control when he indulged in his "drug." When he wasn't "high" on "new relationship energy," Alex was an empathic and attentive partner. "It wasn't like I could just be satisfied with two or three women and settle down. There was never enough, and I was always tempted by the next one. Dawn was okay with us dating and becoming intimate with other women; she enjoyed it up to a point, but she didn't really want to live with another person. Cheryl did end up moving in with us, and it worked out fine for Dawn—the two of them loved it—but I was relieved when Cheryl hooked up with our friend Oscar and went to live with him." Alex's high-

level communication skills, team spirit, and playful creativity made him
a natural for polyamory, but his addictive behavior sabotaged him every
time. Alex, like Thelma, finally joined Sex and Love Addicts Anonymous
(SLAA). Similarly to its sister Twelve Step groups, Alcoholics Anonymous
and Narcotics Anonymous, SLAA preaches abstinence (which in this case
means monogamy rather than celibacy).

At one point, when Alex was having difficulty staying on the wagon, I
suggested that it might be easier if he stayed out of "bars," but he and
Dawn so enjoyed the relaxed openness of poly friendly venues and the
deep friendships they'd established that they continued to gravitate toward
this community and eventually succeeded in establishing better boundaries.

While I've seen too much evidence that sexual addiction is as real as any
other addiction to deny its existence, I've also observed that those who are
the quickest to point the finger at others often have a tendency toward sex
addiction themselves. I usually tell people that if they must have an addiction, sex, along with meditation, hatha yoga, and jogging, are relatively
healthy ones in which to indulge. Sex itself is good for you, and great sex is
very good for you, but the more euphoric and ecstatic the experience, the
more temptation there can be to sell one's soul to the devil. In my circles,
people often joke about "meditation as medication," and many spiritual
teachers are now warning about the dangers of transitory transcendental
states and experiences derailing the attainment of a more abiding but ordinary union with the Divine.

For Tanya, the allure of mind-blowing sex capable of transporting her to
other realms kept her involved in a polyamorous relationship in which she
resented being "a secondary" with none of the privileges, power, or status
of a "primary partner." Tanya is a mature, introspective woman in her
early sixties. She initially consulted me with a complaint about her lover's
wife, Sheila. Her lover, Jerry, was in an open marriage when they met, and
Tanya accepted this but objected to his spending every weekend with his
wife, Sheila, because she "requires a sex partner every weekend, all weekend. Sheila has at least three other lovers besides him, and he's fine with
that, but I'm not. For Sheila, it's all about her getting what she wants, and
she wants virtually all of it. And we're talking his money as well."

Tanya was in a quandary because "Jerry has a loving affectionate heart,
is highly sexed, and is totally present for me when I'm with him. What
happens between us in the bedroom is profound. Last month, I went to a

celestial plane of consciousness—a whole new level for me! He calls me often (but not often enough), tells me he loves me, brings me gifts, and is generally very accepting and easy to talk to, although certain subjects make him bristle. This is hands down the best relationship I've ever had. I'm really happy to have him in my life, but I guess I'm getting jealous."

Tanya easily accepted my coaching to forget about Sheila's issues and concentrate on her own but was less able to hear my warning that she could be in for a rough ride if she thought this relationship was going to be about Jerry meeting her emotional needs. Some months later, Tanya was devastated when Jerry began neglecting her for a new woman. "Is it really a reflection on my self-worth, value, and dignity if he jumps into bed with so many other women while professing so much love for me?" she wondered. "I can open my heart to loads of men, quite deeply, and yes, that often makes me drawn to them sexually, but I don't have to sleep with them all. But maybe I shouldn't be so fast to cast the first stone here; if the right person came along, I might want to do the same thing. But this is hurting me. I know I'm doing it to myself, but I still haven't gotten over it. He just left me in the dust when a new woman came along. He gave her more time than he ever gave me; he was thoughtless, almost cruel. And when she dumped him, he came back to me. I took a breather and then opened the door again. He has never apologized. I have trust issues to begin with, and I'm pretty clear he has Asperger's, and that doesn't help because whenever I want to talk, he gets defensive, and then his anger kicks in, and then he has to shut down and leave because it takes hours for it to physically subside. So then it always becomes about him, and I never get heard.

"He never got how much he hurt me when he was chasing this other woman, how thoroughly he cast me aside, and that is always sitting underneath. And the little things add up and become bigger than the extraordinary sweetness and loving time we share. I think I could handle his being poly much more easily if it were more a matter of polyfidelity or even somewhat more equal."

Tanya imagines that if only Jerry were not polyamorous, if only she were more of an equal partner or got equal time, everything would be fine. That doesn't sound very likely to me, I tell her, but she continues to confuse herself by trying to make allowances based on the idea that he has a right to be polyamorous and that if she is spiritually correct and understanding enough, she can make it work. Why doesn't she dump him if she's suffering? She's considering it, but the sex is too good, and she's not confident of finding someone else to love.

POLYAMORY AND ASPERGER SYNDROME

Asperger syndrome has been relatively recently recognized as a neurobiological disorder somewhat related to autism but characterized by deficiencies in social skills, difficulties with transitions, and difficulties reading body language and other nonverbal cues. Often there is also acute sensitivity to sounds, sights, tastes, and smells and exceptional skill or talent in a specific area. These people are known both for their eccentricity and for their creativity. Einstein, for example, has often been mentioned as a likely Asperger's candidate. Because of the legendary inability of people with Asperger's to navigate social situations and function well in intimate relationships, I wouldn't have expected to find them gravitating toward polyamory, which, as we have seen, thrives on emotional intelligence and excellent communication skills. Nevertheless, serendipity has brought this connection to my attention. Within the space of one day, I discovered that three different people who I'd been interviewing for this book either had been diagnosed with Asperger's or had a poly lover with Asperger's. Considering that Asperger's is thought to be rather rare, I found that significant. When I started reflecting on people I had known, including some of my own partners, I began to notice a common pattern. I began to suspect that a significant minority of people choosing polyamory have Asperger's traits if not the full-blown syndrome.

I asked one of my interviewees who identified himself as having Asperger's how he would account for polyamory and Asperger's being such unlikely bedfellows. His opinion, based on his own life experience, was that Asperger's leads to a technical and strategic way of consciously thinking that is applied to relationships as well as other areas of life. Okay, I thought, so polyamory is more strategic? Perhaps it could be, but only for those of very high intelligence.

Tanya, who suspected that her partner Jerry had Asperger's, directed me to Dr. Amy Marsh, a sex therapist specializing in working with Asperger syndrome (or Aspies as they are affectionately nicknamed). She told me that she had studied Aspies and sexuality for her doctoral research and found that a number were involved in polyamorous relationships. Why?

She guessed that "Aspies gravitate toward intimate situations where there are rules, mutual agreements, parameters, defined roles, and ways to manage their own limited capacities for emotional engagement but still enjoy intimacy (mostly on their terms). . . . My sense is that Aspies will be among those who approach these things in a more formal way than others." She mentioned polyamory as one of several other intimate structures that have this kind of appeal.

This explanation seems to be in line with the strategic thinking concept, but I have another hypothesis. Because Aspies are fairly clueless about social norms and prone to misread or overlook negative reactions to social deviations, they are less likely to be bound by mononormative relationship expectations and more willing to experiment with out of the box arrangements. They don't automatically reject polyamory as socially incorrect as some might do. Instead, they take an unbiased, objective look and decide it may meet their needs. And then they're not bothered by social ostracism because they either don't notice or are used to it because of their other odd behaviors. Additionally, polyamory may make intimate relationships more manageable for them if their partners can meet their own needs for empathy and emotional closeness, which the Aspie may find bewildering elsewhere.

Marsh's description of her love affair with Michael Rossman, best known for his role in the Free Speech movement in the 1960s, illustrates the ways in which polyamory can enable Aspies to succeed at intimacy.[5] Michael Rossman wrote eloquently about his lifelong quest for Oneness, a quest that included numerous spiritual traditions, psychedelics, and sexual encounters, and it was his writing that initially attracted Marsh, who relates that their meeting took place not so long before his death in 2009. "It was kind of like waltzing with a Cyrano de Bergerac, but without the sword," she says. She writes in the third person about one of their encounters:

"The woman lets herself into the flat, climbing stairs that are partially obstructed by papers, rocks, plants, and other natural history specimens. She looks nice. She's dressed in anticipation of meeting her lover, but her clothes don't seem to matter much to him. She can hear the click of his keyboard as she reaches the top of the stairs. A huge piece of printing equipment partially blocks the way to his room, along with stacks of magazines, books, and slippery plastic bags on the floor. She puts her purse on the unmade bed, which is also stacked with books, magazines, newspapers, and mail. Rubber bands lurk in the bedding. The man in the room is lit by the computer monitor, still typing on his keyboard. His long gray ponytail hangs down his back. He does not turn around; he does not acknowledge her entrance to the room. She will have to wait, as always, for him to make the transition from one activity to another.

"Eventually the man turns to the woman with a greeting, spends a few more minutes at the keyboard, then gets up from his chair and beckons her into the kitchen with a crisp command. She follows. She expects tea first and then some conversation as he sorts a month's worth of vitamins and supplements into various compartmentalized lidded boxes. Or perhaps tonight he'll be scraping grease from his stovetop with a razor or delicately removing the last bits of dried flesh from a rat skeleton (many small skeletons and natural history specimens gather dust in his flat). Manual activity seems to accompany his shift into sociable interaction. Their conversation is lively, interesting, but for all its warmth is never sentimental and seldom addresses emotions. It is not a 'lover-like' exchange. Unlike other lovers, these two never indulge in mutual reminiscences designed to renew emotional closeness after a separation. Almost everything that has happened between them, good or bad, is never mentioned between them again. To the woman, this feels strange."

Switching back to the first person, Marsh continues, "I had some struggles with the way things were going. I really yearned for a dollop of fuzzy affection now and then. . . . Eventually we got to the point where we could detect each other's deliberate subtle body movements. Without giving a sign through any corresponding physical movement, I would send the energy streaming as a gentle rain; the brush of leaves; something heavy, light, swirling around the shoulders or going straight to the heart. These were sometimes mere micromovements of intention. The man before me would gasp, shudder, widen his eyes, and so I knew I'd hit my mark.

"It was pleasurable in the extreme. It was lovely, entrancing. Gleeful and fascinating. It encompassed merging and separation. It was profoundly sexual. I wouldn't say it was orgasmic, though, because it never peaked like that. . . . From the beginning, I had struggled with the very strange, frustrating, and unsatisfactory features of this relationship—features which were seemingly so much at odds with the closeness we'd achieved in the subtle realm. It took a few months before the 'what if it's Asperger syndrome' lightbulb lit up, and once it did, Michael was both amused by my great efforts to understand him and understandably resistant to attempts to label him. As time went on, however, I believe he came to understand

certain aspects of his life and relationships as a story that included neuro-
logical difference (over and above a glancing embrace of ADD [attention
deficit disorder]). He as much as said it, near the end."

Marsh recalls that Michael Rossman's wife, unaware that Michael was
an Aspie, took his relational deficits personally, as the "neurotypical" partner is likely to do. He took very literally their vows at their commitment
ceremony, which included openness and sexual freedom. She went along
with it, hoping he'd change. And he, because he'd been perfectly honest from the beginning, in front of all their friends, couldn't understand
her hurt and jealousy. "That's another thing about Aspies," Marsh says,
"it's kind of written in stone for them, and it can be a lot of work to get a
renegotiation going!" That's why she thinks a lot of work has to be done
up front via agreements and parameters to succeed in any kind of Aspie
relationship. "Be very careful what you include," she warns, "because it's
not easily undone."[6]

POLYAMORY AS A STABILIZING FORCE

Sex and love addiction can traumatize an addict's partners, and to the
extent that partners fit the codependency profile, polyamory can effectively skirt the need to face an addiction and the painful feelings it covers.
However, polyamory can also be utilized as a healthy means of coping with
psychological difficulties, preexisting trauma, differences in sexual desire,
and the garden-variety erotic boredom so common in long-term monogamous marriages.

Esther Perel, a Manhattan couples therapist, wisely advises that "the
presence of the third is a fact of life; how we deal with it is up to us. We
can approach it with fear, avoidance, and moral outrage; or we can bring
to it a robust curiosity and a sense of intrigue. . . . Acknowledging the third
has to do with validating the erotic separateness of your partner. It follows
that our partner's sexuality does not belong to us. It isn't just for and about
us, and we should not assume that it rightfully falls within our jurisdiction.
It doesn't. . . . Accommodating the third opens up an erotic expanse where
eros needn't worry about wilting. In that expanse, we can be deeply moved
by our partner's otherness, and soon thereafter deeply aroused."[7]

Perel suggests that "we view monogamy not as a given but as a choice. As
such it becomes a negotiated decision. More to the point, if we're planning

to spend fifty years with one soul—and we want a happy jubilee—it may be wise to review our contract at various junctures. Just how accommodating each couple may be to the third varies. But at least a nod is more apt to sustain desire with our one and only over the long haul—perhaps even to create a new 'art of loving' for the twenty-first century couple."[8]

Robert Masters is a Canadian therapist who formerly headed an intentional community called Xanthyros, which utilized many radical measures to help people awaken to their divinity, including nonmonogamy. From what I've heard from friends who spent time there, polyamory was a very effective means of penetrating the personality, similar to its use in earlier spiritual groups. Since this community disbanded some years ago, Masters has changed his views. He now believes that "if we were to put monogamy up against polyamory, with regard to depth, awakening potential, and capacity for real intimacy, which would come out on top? Monogamy, by a landslide, so long as we're talking about mature monogamy, as opposed to conventional (or growth-stunting and passion-dulling) monogamy, referred to from now on as immature monogamy. Immature monogamy is, especially in men, frequently infected with promiscuous desire and fantasy, however much that might be repressed or camouflaged with upstanding virtues. Airbrush this, infuse it with talk of integrity and unconditional love and jealousy-transcending ethics, consider bringing in another partner or two, and you're closer than near to polyamorous or multiple-partnering territory."[9]

Masters came to his appreciation for monogamy relatively late in life after fully immersing himself in multiple partner relating. While he does not emphasize stability as a criterion for preferring monogamy, I get the feeling that this is part of its current appeal for him. Instead, Masters uses the language of attachment and critiques multipartner relating as a way to avoid attachment. In my experience, it doesn't. True, plenty of people use multipartner relating as a strategy to avoid attachment (some even recommend this), but in my experience, attachment is a powerful force that can override any mental argument or situational defense. Many people hope to find greater stability, depth, and personal growth in their intimate relating by choosing polyamory, while others seek the same qualities in monogamy. The bottom line is that, whether we like it or not, all relationships are dynamic by nature, and any effort to avoid this reality is doomed to failure.

While there are no data to support the common assumption that polyamory impairs attachment or is risky to the longevity of a pair bond—and, in fact, Perel and others acknowledge that it may be just the opposite—I suspect that whether polyamory or monogamy does more to stabilize a relationship depends on the individuals involved and their life experience. When two or more people are well matched, opening their relationship usually makes it stronger. When they're not, opening up can be destabilizing. Neither monogamy nor polyamory has a corner on immaturity, and people can gravitate toward both from a position of maturity or its opposite. In a recent conversation, Robert agreed with me that this is so but felt that few evolved people would want to engage with more than one regardless of the quality of the relationships.

The following excerpt from a dialogue with a couple working on their issues about sexual exclusivity with spiritual teacher Byron Katie (who prefers monogamy for herself) illustrates how being open to what is, rather than trying to impose a concept of what one believes, may be the best way to settle this question.[10]

Ellen: I am frustrated with Charlie because he's in love with another woman. He's been having affairs for fifteen years. I can only be with him if I accept that he has an affair running. I want Charlie to realize what he's doing and stop thinking that it's normal to be in a very close relationship and still have an affair.

Katie: So sweetheart, "You need him to be monogamous"—is that true? Or "You want him to be monogamous"—is that true?

Ellen: No. I think I will get bored.

Katie: So he has the perfect partner, and you have the perfect partner. How do you react when you believe this thought "I want him to be monogamous," and he hasn't been—for fifteen years?

Ellen: I get really frustrated. I try all kinds of things. I try to be open and nice and say okay, do it, and then I hide my jealousy. Or I have tantrums and scream and try different ways to manipulate him.

Katie: So does that thought bring peace or stress into your life—"I want him to be monogamous"?

Ellen: Stress.

Katie: So "I want him to be monogamous"—turn it around.

Ellen: I don't want him to be monogamous.

Katie: Now give me an example of why your life is better because he's not monogamous.

Ellen: I have many! Okay, it keeps me on the track of watching myself and my thoughts. I don't get bored. He comes back much more loving.

Katie: Now why is *his* life better because he's not monogamous? Reasons that you're thankful for. The things that you like about it in his life. Advantages to *him* that really are advantages to *you*.

Ellen: Oh. He doesn't get bored with me.

Katie: Yes, when he's gone, you're not arguing.

Katie: Because *his* life is not monogamous, and that's how he's living it. He does what he has been doing for fifteen years, and you have continued to accept him back into your life and that tells me that it is okay with you that he isn't monogamous and you're fooling yourself, lying to both of you, when you say that it isn't okay, and that is the pain that you both feel.

Katie (To Charlie): Why do you need more than one woman, in your relationship with her for fifteen years? Why do you prefer non-monogamy?

Charlie: It's more fun.

Katie (to Ellen): So look into his eyes, honey. You wanted to know. So there is his answer.

Charlie: And there's more. I find that there's something. . . . I feel like when I limit myself to one woman, I feel like I'm in a box. . . . It's almost like it doesn't feel like love to say that I'm just with one woman. I feel that if I deny myself being open with other people, and that includes sexually . . . , I'm denying something that's quite natural in me. And I tried monogamy, and it didn't work for me. I noticed that I punished the woman that I was with, for me not being able to live the life that I wanted to live, I blamed her for the decisions I was making.

The simple but structured format[11] that Byron Katie uses to help people stop arguing with reality and make peace with whatever is happening whether or not they ultimately decide to change things may sound a little odd to those unfamiliar with it. However, it's a very useful tool that can be applied in many situations to resolve both inner and outer conflict. In this case, it quickly moves Ellen out of her unquestioned assumption that she wants her partner to be monogamous and brings her to the realization that while she's been resisting nonmonogamy, it's only her resistance and fear that are causing her to struggle. When she opens her mind and gives up the struggle, it becomes apparent that, on the whole, she likes having a nonmonogamous partner, even though she is apparently monogamous herself because it makes for a livelier, more interesting relationship with more opportunities for personal growth.

Psychologist David Ley has studied couples in which the wives are nonmonogamous with the approval and encouragement of their often monogamous husbands. His 2009 book *Insatiable Wives*[12] offers evidence that those who practice nonmonogamy tend to have extremely effective communication skills and relationship skills and are no more or no less pathological than any other group. Some of the husbands enjoyed vicariously experiencing the sexuality of other men and welcomed the opportunity to explore their bisexuality from a safe distance. In chapter 8, we'll discuss how polyamory can provide a context for people to directly explore bisexuality or to dip a toe in the forbidden waters of homosexuality or heterosexuality depending on their existing identity. Ley points out that many of the things that make polyamory exciting and compelling are linked to biological, neurochemical, and evolutionary processes that underlie human behavior. For example, "The biological effects of sperm competition [discussed in chapter 10 of this book] and other evolutionary mechanisms that were intended to prevent or control the risk of cuckoldry are being subverted by couples in a fashion they use to reignite and maintain high levels of sexual excitement within their marriages,"[13] according to Ley.

One woman he interviewed put it this way: "I've never met anyone I respect and love more than [my husband]. So it's not about seeking something that's missing. It's about added fun and enjoyment. It keeps our sex more alive, because it's not the same, it's broken up, variety in between. I think that's one of the reasons why sex is just off the charts for us."[14]

MANAGING TRAUMA, INTENSITY, AND UNEQUAL SEX DRIVES

Keeping erotic love alive and maintaining a healthy sense of separateness motivates some long-term couples to adopt polyamory. Both singles and couples often enjoy the greater intensity of having multiple partners. Polyamory can also serve singles who find exclusivity to be an emotional challenge, especially in the early stages of relationship when trust, compatibility, and commitment are still being tested. Dane's reflections illustrate all these motivations.[15]

Dane is a tall, slender man in his mid-thirties. Everything about him is intense, including his sexuality. "In some ways I prefer monogamy," Dane admits, "and right now I'm mostly monogamous, but most of the dating world doesn't have time for the deep one-on-one cocoons I enjoy, so it's easier to find lovers if I don't require so much undivided attention with me. The first woman I explored open relationship with noticed she was opening up to me more than she had to any other man, in part because she didn't feel on the spot and had a back door herself. Some women have time enough but get overwhelmed by the energetic intensity that deep communication and lovemaking often brings. I discovered when I had more than one lover my sex drive increased due to the wonderful feeling of being wanted by two or three women rather than being overwhelming for one woman. It's a real turn-off for me to have energy to give that a partner has no room to receive, which would happen for me 90 percent of the time in a monogamous relationship, simply because I prefer more intensity and have a lot of time and energy I enjoy investing in relationships."

Dr. Ley, who specializes in treating trauma, believes that in some cases nonmonogamy is not a symptom of trauma or emotional disturbance but may actually be an adaptive mechanism that allows individuals to overcome effects of trauma and loss. He feels that one of his interviewees who was abused as a child was able to have a truly intimate emotional relationship only in a polyamorous framework. He suggests that monogamy was simply too threatening and restrictive for her to tolerate emotionally.

Psychologist Peter Thomas emphasizes the importance of developing an internal working model of an effective protector in order to establish and maintain healthy boundaries, a crucial developmental step that is often missed in adults with a history of childhood abuse.[16] As a result, these individuals can be easily retraumatized in polyamorous relating because they tend to dissociate and become passive when they feel threatened, making them easy prey for the sexual predators who sometimes show up at sexually open gatherings as well as becoming victims of well-meaning but insensitive partners. However, they can also benefit from interacting with a committed partner who is caring, nurturing, and protective without being possessive. In a committed polyamorous relationship, adults who are recovering from childhood abuse can reap the benefits of developing trust in the reliable protector they missed as children and eventually develop this protective agency within themselves.

Alex and Janet Lessin are a good example of a couple who are committed to the practice of polyamory as one tool in healing the wounds from Janet's childhood sexual abuse. Shortly after Janet and Alex got together about ten years ago, Alex arranged an evening with another couple who'd been his longtime lovers. Janet took to Altheia right away but experienced an intense revulsion to Hercules. Earlier that day, she'd learned that her mother was dying but decided to go ahead with the date that meant so much to Alex. Later that evening, Alex, a professional therapist who'd trained in holotropic breathwork with Dr. Stan Grof and G-spot massage with Charles Muir, was using these techniques with Janet when the long-repressed memory of being orally raped and suffocated at the age of four by her mother's boyfriend, who was bald like Hercules, surfaced. At the time, Janet had left her body and, while presumed dead for more than thirty minutes, observed dispassionately from above while the adults struggled to revive her. She reports that angel-like guides showed her several alternate futures that led to her deciding to remain among the living to protect her mother from prosecution for murder.[17]

Alex subsequently applied all the tools in his therapeutic tool kit, including psychodramatically reenacting the rape while he played a protective father role, to help Janet heal from this and other childhood traumas. He reports that her lifelong aversion to oral sex, along with her distaste for Hercules, eventually dissipated. Because of Janet's unconscious negative associations with bald-headed men, it's unlikely that she would ever have chosen to become intimate with one outside a circumstance like this. Janet's childhood wounds have posed challenges to her ongoing efforts to establish healthy relationships, but with Alex's loyal support, she's overcome many of her fears and enthusiastically embraced polyamory.

DEMOGRAPHICS

There have been two surveys of the American polyamory community and one in the United Kingdom within the past two decades all relying on demographics gathered from self-identified polyamorists who attend events or participate in online discussions about polyamory. In my experience, people who are active in the polyamory community are not necessarily typical of those who are actively polyamorous but choose not to associate themselves with those groups. My impression is that neither the more socially conservative nor the more socially radical individuals are well represented. In addition, people of color, those of lower socioeconomic status, young people, gay men, and, to a lesser extent, lesbian women are underrepresented in the self-proclaimed polyamory community, although I find abundant evidence, both direct and indirect, that these groups are at least as likely to be involved in polyamorous relationships.

Walston[18] distributed a questionnaire via polyamory e-mail lists on the Internet in 1999 and received 430 responses. *Loving More* magazine collected data from 1,000 people attending polyamory conferences in the late 1990s.[19] Barker surveyed thirty poly people via the Internet in the United Kingdom, Europe, and the United States.[20] All these studies report similar results, except that Barker's sample was almost entirely bisexual, and the motivations they identified are essentially the same as those put forth by those whose interviews I've shared here. Walston reported that more than half the respondents reported that their reasons for practicing polyamory included openness and honesty, personal growth, personal freedom, sexual variety, romantic variety, philosophical ideal, sense of community, and needs not being met by one relationship. Fewer than half the respondents gave these motivators: protest against cultural norms, falling in love, additional adults to help with child rearing, economic reasons, partner falling in love, and other unnamed reasons. Interestingly, the only significant gender difference was that women were more likely than men or transsexuals to say that they had chosen polyamory because of falling in love.

Both surveys found that polyamorists were more highly educated than the general public and that the majority were no longer identified with the religion in which they were raised, although most had some spiritual affiliation. Both also reported a high incidence of bisexuality, although nearly 30 percent of the *Loving More* respondents didn't identify their sexual orientation at all. The *Loving More* survey found that while individuals had incomes comparable to the national median, 78 percent of households were way above the national median for households, and more than a quarter reported six-digit household incomes, although only 44 percent were married, and only 20 percent were in live-in poly relationships. I suspect that the high household incomes are more likely influenced by high numbers of affluent two-career professional couples than the combined incomes of three or more wage earners, but both factors probably contribute. Walston did not inquire about income but found that 16 percent lived with three or more partners, while 30 percent lived alone, and more than half were married or cohabiting couples.

Eighty percent of those who completed the *Loving More* survey admitted that they had experienced jealousy, a topic not included in the Walston report, and 93 percent were concerned about discrimination against polys, with 43 percent reporting that they had directly experienced prejudice, although only 17 percent had gotten negative responses after coming out to spouses, with lower percentages of negative response from others. Almost all the respondents in both studies had come out to their partners, and most who had children were also out to their children but were less likely to tell parents, employers, and neighbors.

We still have very little data on the demographics, motivations, and concerns of polyamorous people, not to mention the incidence of polyamory in the general population, although extrapolations from the *Loving More* data estimate that one out of every 500 adults in the United States is polyamorous. Others have speculated that something like 3.5 percent of the adult population prefer polyamorous relationships, which would put the figure at about 10 million, but I predict that by the time a large-scale survey is undertaken, this figure will be found to be much higher.

3

THE HISTORY OF POLYAMORY

There is little question that while nonmonogamy has been prominent in most cultures throughout time, polyamory in its modern form emerged in the United States. Although its roots go back to the utopian communities of the nineteenth century, responsible nonmonogamy began to grow vigorously in the turmoil of the sexual revolution of the 1970s. Twenty-first-century polyamory is quite different from these early experiments, but we can understand its origins and evolution by examining its history.

ONEIDA AND COMPLEX MARRIAGE

The best known of the nineteenth-century utopian communities is the Oneida Community, founded by John Humphrey Noyes in 1848. Oneida grew to 300 members in its heyday before abandoning the doctrine of complex marriage under legal pressure. In 1881, Oneida morphed to a corporate enterprise, Oneida Limited, which continues to this day as a successful silverware company. Noyes, who came from a privileged upper-class background, adopted a number of unorthodox beliefs and practices while studying for the ministry at Yale Divinity School. He later married Harriet Holton, a wealthy and well-connected woman whose support, along with that of his own family, helped establish the community in upstate New York.

The Oneida Community was a spiritual community that, following the example of the earliest Christians, held all property in common and attempted to overcome traditional gender roles. The most controversial aspect of the whole infamous project was the doctrine of complex marriage. In complex marriage, all the men and all the women within the community were considered married to each other. Even couples who were already married when joining the community were required to have separate rooms and open their marriage to others. No two people could have exclusive attachment with each other and would be separated and not allowed to see each other for a certain length of time if this were suspected. Men were required to withhold ejaculation during intercourse unless conception was intended, and more mature members of the community were given the task of initiating the younger ones into sexual and spiritual practices.

Oneidans felt that achieving perfection and living without sin required that they abandon traditional marriage. Noyes believed that the spiritual dimension of sex brought partners closer to God as well as each other. "The new commandment is that we love one another, not by pairs, as in the world, but en masse," he decreed.[1]

In theory, complex marriage eliminated jealousy and possessiveness by marrying all the men of the community to all the women and encouraging members to enjoy frequent lovemaking and multiple partners. The strategy of managing jealousy through creating an abundance of partners has continued to be used into the twenty-first century with varying degrees of success, as we will see in future chapters. Oneida men took responsibility for birth control by withholding ejaculation, which was intended to provide Oneida women with greater sexual satisfaction and fewer pregnancies than their contemporaries. This in itself was a huge departure from Victorian standards, which did not support women taking pleasure in sex at all.

Although I have not been able to discover a direct link between Noyes and Tantric teachings, it's interesting to note that his spiritual doctrine of perfectionism, his emphasis on the sacredness of sexuality, and the sexual practice of nonejaculation for men can all be found in ancient Tantric teachings. Is it a coincidence that many modern-day American polyamorists also mix inclusive love with Tantric teachings?

Despite its shortcomings, Oneida was so far ahead of its time that it's continued to be a model for polyamorous innovators to the present day. Twenty-first-century polyamorists have been less inspired by another early experiment in multiple partner marriage that adhered more closely to the patriarchal tradition of polygamy for men only and emphasized traditional sex roles and conservative values. Nevertheless, HBO's popular *Big Love* series is based on the spiritual heirs of Mormon prophet Joseph Smith, who had thirty-three wives and set the precedent for nearly all the elders of the early Church of Jesus Christ of Latter-Day Saints (LDS) to follow in his footsteps.

MORMON POLYGAMY

Joseph Smith's teachings on celestial or patriarchal marriage, which have come to be known as the Mormon Doctrine of Plural Wives, arose in the 1840s. The doctrine was not officially announced until 1852 by Smith's successor Brigham Young in a special conference of the elders of the LDS. Although polygamy had its detractors even among the faithful, it was widely practiced until officially rejected as Mormon doctrine under federal pressure as a condition for Utah's statehood. Even today, it's estimated that 30,000 to 60,000 renegade practitioners still adhere to this form of group marriage, which seems to hold a fascination for many people.

Both Oneida and the LDS church are thought to have been influenced by an earlier Christian preacher named Jacob Cochran,[2] who advocated a practice he called *spiritual wifery*, along with communal ownership of property, as early as 1818. Cochran did not consider traditional marriage valid and instead assigned and often shifted couplings as he saw fit, with many of the women paired with him at one time or another. Even though Cochran stayed with the couple concept, his innovations with mix-and-match dyads were too scandalous for nineteenth-century New England, and he was soon imprisoned for lewdness, lascivious behavior, and adultery. After his release from prison, he founded a new community in New York State from which many members were later converted by Mormon missionaries.

BROOK FARM COMMUNITY

New England in the early 1800s was a hotbed of social, philosophical, and cultural dissent. The downside of the industrial revolution was becoming apparent to the intelligentsia, who were eager to explore health-promoting lifestyles. In addition to the previously described communities, New England spawned the Transcendentalist movement, which involved

well-known literary figures such as Ralph Waldo Emerson, Henry David
Thoreau, Margaret Fuller, Nathaniel Hawthorne, and Walt Whitman and
was closely linked with another utopian community named Brook Farm.

Started in 1841 by Unitarian minister, Harvard graduate, and social
reformer George Ripley and his wife Sophia, with author Nathaniel Hawthorne as one of the original trustees, Brook Farm was initially conceived
as an agrarian cooperative that would provide its members a more natural
and wholesome lifestyle. Ripley, as well as Emerson, is known to have had
large libraries that included European writers as well as translations of
Indian and Chinese classics. It's possible that John Noyes may have been
exposed to Tantric and Taoist philosophies through this group, although
their own departures from traditional marital and gender roles were less
regimented and kept in the background and out of the headlines.

In 1844, Albert Brisbane, who translated the works of French utopian
philosopher Charles Fourier into English during his frequent visits to
Brook Farm, convinced the directors to become a Fourierist community.
Fourier's ideas are now largely forgotten, although they reached a wide
audience in the United States in the 1840s through Brisbane's columns in
the *New York Tribune*.

In addition to his very detailed prescriptions for the physical structures
and agricultural, business, and social organization of these communes, or
phalansteries, as he called them, Fourier held some unusual views on the
subject of monogamy. Fourier asserted that a harmonious society required
an awareness of the "laws of passionate attraction." He believed that each
person has a set capacity for the number of lovers he or she can engage
with at one time, with a range from zero to eight. Both ends of the spec-
trum were thought to be quite rare, with most people naturally falling
somewhere in the middle.[3] Fourier also took a strong stance on the importance of pleasure and sexual gratification and was an advocate of women's
rights, gay rights, and sexual freedom long before the sexual revolutions of
the twentieth century dawned.

EMMA GOLDMAN, FREE LOVE, AND THE
FIRST WAVE OF THE SEXUAL REVOLUTION

Emma Goldman was one of my earliest heroines. A feminist anarchist who
devoted her life to organizing support for the independence of women at

a time when women in the United States had not yet won the right to vote and when advocating access to birth control was grounds for imprisonment, she was also a passionate supporter of free love. While the scope of her work was not limited to women's issues, Goldman is often credited with bringing sexual liberty and reproductive rights into serious political conversation.

In the early nineteenth century, the term *free love*, whose creation is attributed to Oneida founder John Noyes, carried a different meaning than it took on in the 1960s. Originally, it implied freedom for women from the ownership of men through the institution of marriage. The Oneidan version of free love could be likened to today's term *polyfidelity* (which refers to a type of closed group marriage), but Goldman and her fellow anarchists didn't believe in imposing any kind of structure or rules on the free flow of love. It is this meaning of freedom from legislation or mental constructs, as well as equality for all genders, that inspired my own vision for polyamory as a more heartfelt way to love. It seems ironic that some polyamorous people, as well as monogamous nonheterosexuals, are now clamoring to have their marriages recognized by church and state.

A talented orator and writer as well as a nurse midwife, Goldman had an impact on Western culture that wasn't fully recognized until long after her death in 1940. She was also ruthlessly honest in revealing her struggle with jealousy arising from sharing her beloved. Her gift for formulating and articulating a critique of patriarchal values gave rise to changes that are still unfolding in the twenty-first century. In 1930, Goldman wrote, "I demand the independence of woman, her right to support herself; to live for herself; to love whomever she pleases, or as many as she pleases. I demand freedom for both sexes, freedom of action, freedom in love and freedom in motherhood."[4]

Emma Goldman, like Victoria Woodhull, another early feminist and free love advocate, did more than theorize about free love. Both women boldly exercised their right to love whomever they pleased at a time when even monogamous sexually active unmarried women were considered sluts. Woodhull is even known to have openly engaged in triadic love relationships, including one with a prominent Christian minister that caused a national scandal.[5]

Politically and emotionally, Goldman, the quintessential anarchist who thought that voting was a waste of time, and Woodhull, the first woman to run for the presidency of the United States in 1872, were worlds apart, but both created many effective cocreative partnerships with men that merged their intimate and professional needs. This model for harnessing the power of sexual passion in service of social goals is a theme elaborated on a generation later by other key figures in the evolution of polyamory.

SCIENCE FICTION AND THE CHURCH OF ALL WORLDS

If there is any one book that can be said to have kicked off the present-day evolution of polyamory, that book would have to be Robert Heinlein's *Stranger in a Strange Land*. This novel, with a Martian-raised human hero who finds the concept of sexual possessiveness very peculiar and starts a religion based on sharing, struck a deep chord with the millions who've read it since its publication in 1961. Heinlein wrote many other science-fiction novels with polyamorous themes that continue to be widely read today, though none has achieved the popularity of *Stranger in a Strange Land*.

Polyamory as a model or support system for creating transformation in the larger culture has been a popular topic with many science-fiction and fantasy writers, such as Thea Alexander, Marion Zimmer Bradley, Ernest Callenbach, Spider Robinson, Starhawk, and John Varley. Consensual multipartner relationships have also figured prominently in the books of literary giants such as Anais Nin, Doris Lessing, and Alice Walker.

I vaguely remember reading *Stranger in a Strange Land* as a freshman in college in 1969 and finding it delightful but not earthshaking. Perhaps it did seep into my subconscious mind and influence my future career unbeknownst to me. When I reread it about twenty years later, I was shocked by the sexist language and dialogue that had slipped right across my prefeminist radar. Why, I wondered, was this particular book so influential? We may never be able to fully answer that question, but some portion of its impact may have to do with neopagan leader Oberon Zell. When I first met Oberon, or Otter as he was called at the time, in the 1980s, he had long since founded the Church of All Worlds (CAW) and was publisher of *Green Egg Magazine*, an early neopagan periodical. He and his wife Morning Glory had been in a triad for some years with the magazine's editor and were later to form a group marriage with three others that incorporated many of Heinlein's ideas.

CAW itself was inspired by and based on *Stranger in a Strange Land*, and the Zells, who invented the term *polyamory* in 1990, have done much to spread these beliefs among the pagan community in the United States. Oberon asserts that "polyamory has really caught on as a primary relationship model for the younger generation, especially in the worldwide pagan community which is estimated at ten million adherents and still growing. In the Pagan community, polyamory is so well accepted as an option— even an ideal—that those of us who engage in it don't even merit a raised eyebrow. Far from being seen as scandalous (as would have been the case prior to the '60s), flamboyantly polyamorous folk such as ourselves are looked upon as models. . . . At this time, there is scarcely any Pagan group anywhere in the world that doesn't have some connection with some other group(s) through lover relationships between them."[6]

According to the Zells, the principle here is exactly the same as the medieval custom of "fostering" children out to be raised in other households and of royalty marrying princes or princesses of different nationalities. The idea is to forge bonds and alliances based on personal relationships. Oberon believes that "polyamory will continue to grow and spread throughout the world. It's a viral meme with an extremely high promulgation factor! The Vision that we have, and which you articulated so well in that article you wrote back in 1990, is of a world-wide new culture permeated beneath the surface by a vast network of lovers. When it's necessary to pull together a team project of some sort—whether something so simple as moving to a new home, or something so large as creating a new organization—or even a movement—lovers are the ones you can best count on to show up and get involved. This is how MG and I have managed to accomplish pretty much everything we've done in our lives—by having a wide pool of diversely-talented lovers to tap to become involved."[7]

CAW is the pagan group most identified with polyamory, and while I must emphasize that *all* pagans are not polyamorous, CAW is not alone. For example, Starhawk, who is known in some quarters as the witch whose appointment to the faculty of a Catholic University got Matthew Fox, renegade priest and creator of the Macro Cosmic Mass, excommunicated has written many well respected books on witchcraft and ritual. Rather than modeling her organization on a novel, Starhawk created her own fictional world featuring polyamorous relationships as a basis for social change movements in her first novel, *The Fifth Sacred Thing*.[8]

ROBERT RIMMER

Robert Rimmer is another author whose novels played a huge role in inspiring modern-day polyamory. His best-selling *Harrad Experiment* was first published in 1966 and, along with Heinlein's *Stranger in a Strange Land*, influenced a whole generation of young people to question monogamy as an ideal and to create their own experiments in group marriage. *Harrad Experiment* described an undergraduate program designed to liberate students from sexual repression and monogamous conditioning and teach them to embrace healthy open relating. It eventually sold nearly 3 million copies and still evokes fond memories among many baby boomers who have long since forgotten exactly what it was all about.

Harrad was followed by a series of other widely read novels, including *Proposition 31*, which explored group marriage and its legalization; *Thursday My Love*, which addressed extramarital sex; and *Come Live My Life*, which bears an uncanny resemblance to a recent reality TV show about mate swapping (as in living in another household, not a sexual one-night stand). All of Rimmer's writing emphasizes the importance of integrating sex, love, and spirituality and maintaining high ethical standards even while struggling with typical human fears and difficult emotions.

One of his later novels, *The Immoral Reverend* (1985), features a polyamorous Unitarian minister from the Boston area who starts a sex-positive church, not unlike some of the nineteenth-century efforts discussed earlier in this chapter. And, in fact, the Unitarian Universalist Church was the first mainstream religious institution to officially welcome polyamorists into its ranks.

Rimmer, who died in 2001 at the age of eighty-four, was a tireless crusader for saner family structures until the end of his days. He was no literary giant, but he was a masterful storyteller and popular speaker on the college and social science lecture circuit. Rimmer refused to disclose anything about his personal life until the deaths of the couple that he and Erma, his wife for almost sixty years, were intimate with allowed him to talk freely.

I doubt that anyone was shocked to learn that the Rimmers had participated in a long-term relationship with another couple and that this relationship was a model for many of his fictionalized accounts of group marriage. In his miniautobiography, included in the Twenty-Fifth Anniversary Edition of *Harrad*, Bob Rimmer also discusses his military service in India in World War II, where he was first exposed to Tantric teachings on the sacredness of sexuality. While polyamory and Tantra do not have to go together, Rimmer's writings have planted many seeds.

After we'd corresponded for several years, I finally met Bob and Erma Rimmer face-to-face in the early 1990s in Rowe, Massachusetts, where Ryam Nearing and I had convened the first East Coast Loving More Conference. It was Bob who encouraged Ryam and me to join forces and replace our separate newsletters with *Loving More* magazine. Additionally, Bob generously shipped me copies of all his out-of-print books, which I made available as a lending library before used books could be easily located on the Internet. Bob also supported the revival of the Kirkridge Conferences in the early 1990s, bringing me into contact with an earlier generation of love, sex, and intimacy activists based on the East Coast.

THE SECOND AMERICAN SEXUAL REVOLUTION

I came of age in the midst of the sexual revolution heralded by *Time* magazine in 1964 and pronounced dead by *Time* in 1984, a casualty of AIDS, an economic downturn, and/or the radical right, depending on whom you ask. The year 1984 happens to be the same year I found myself beginning the work of organizing today's polyamory movement.

The increasing acceptance of consensual nonmonogamy, open marriage, and other experiments in loving more than one are only one manifestation of the many shifts in sexual values and cultural norms that occurred during those tumultuous twenty years. The sexual revolution as a whole created a climate in which the behaviors that have come to be known as polyamory were able to be seen and experienced by large numbers of people in the Western world for the first time since the rise of the Catholic Church.

Although many people today think of polyamory as a hedonistic, self-centered, and godless approach to love, Christian clergy have been instrumental in breaking the cultural monopoly of monogamy during both the first and the second sexual revolution. As we have seen, many of the nineteenth-century nonmonogamous utopian communities were founded by Christian preachers, and in the mid-twentieth century, Christian clergy again provided much of the spiritual and intellectual underpinnings for validating alternatives to monogamous marriage.

Dr. Robert Francoeur is among the most prolific academic authors to advocate a greater range of sexual and marital choices. After rejecting the celibacy required by the Catholic priesthood, Francouer acquired the distinction of becoming a married Catholic priest after the Vatican granted him permission to wed. He and his wife Anna were among the first to write about changing attitudes toward love and sex as an evolutionary imperative. In their 1974 book *Hot and Cool Sex*,[9] they reexamine the concepts of fidelity, jealousy, and postpatriarchal sex and convincingly portray open marriage as a path to growth.

Bob Francouer was the first of this circle of East Coast Christian clergy to reach out to me in the early 1990s after the publication of my book *Love without Limits*. He introduced me to a well-established network who had been working together toward greater sexual and emotional freedom for both married and single people since the 1960s. Many of them were, like myself, veterans of the sexual revolution, but while I had been a teenage hippie in those days, they were already married and professionally established adults with successful careers when this wave of sexual freedom hit. In those pre-Internet, pre–cell phone, pre–e-mail days, networking depended more on the written word and face-to-face meetings. Bob Rimmer's books were one channel of connection, and the Kirkridge Conferences were another.

I was delighted to connect with an earlier generation of pioneers, such as Dr. Rusty and Della Roy; Dr. Gerald Jud; Reverend Raymond Lawrence, PhD; Sister Annette Covatta, PhD; and Reverend Hal Minor. Gerry Jud in particular, who must have been in his seventies at the time, was very persistent in urging me to come meet with this group of poly clergy, as I dubbed them, at his retreat center in rural Pennsylvania. A Yale graduate and veteran of the civil rights movement, he'd left his position as a church executive many years ago and founded a successful growth center in New York State called Shalom Mountain. By the time we met, he'd moved on to a new venue called Timshel, along with his artist wife and another couple they were courting.

In 1993, Gerry invited me to speak at a wonderful conference held at St. Peter's Church in New York City called "The Union of Sex and Spirit." It seemed like the perfect opportunity to meet a young polyamorous pastor I'd been corresponding with, and it was love at first sight. We ended up sharing the loft in Ray Lawrence's Times Square apartment, climbing over cases of his newly released *Poisoning of Eros*[10] to get into bed. The young pastor was concerned about what would transpire if our relationship ever became public knowledge, but this never happened. However, he was subsequently defrocked after confiding to members of his "open and affirming congregation" (meaning that they accepted nonheterosexual members) that he and his wife were sharing the parish house with their good Christian girlfriend.

The Union of Sex and Spirit event inspired me to later create the Celebration of Eros Conferences on the West Coast and led to my collaboration with the poly clergy network to organize a new series of Kirkridge Conferences that later evolved into the grassroots East Coast organization called The Body Sacred. Gerry Jud once confided to me that twenty years of experience had convinced these very astute activists that sacred sexuality was a far more viable cause and far more palatable to the mainstream culture than nonmonogamy and would eventually lead to similar changes in marital norms. This was one of many reasons I subsequently changed the focus of my own work to Tantra and sexual healing.

Over twenty years earlier, a series of conferences produced by Rustum Roy and his wife Della at the same Christian retreat center had bridged the East Coast–West Coast divide by introducing easterners to one of the best-known experiments of the sexual revolution, Sandstone Retreat, located in the hills above Topanga Canyon in Los Angeles County.

Sandstone was founded by John and Barbara Williamson in 1967, and along with Esalen Institute, Sandstone brought together the concepts of humanistic psychology with sexual freedom. Esalen, which similarly to Brook Farm kept its sex life in the background and later did its best to retreat from the sexual frontier, continues as a successful retreat center. Sandstone, which put much of its focus on open sexuality and extramarital activities, closed its doors in 1972, partly as a result of legal issues.

The Williamsons were profoundly influenced by the work of Dr. Abraham Maslow. Maslow, one of the giants of the humanistic psychology movement, is well known for his theories of human need hierarchies, eupsychian management, and group synergy. Maslow was a fan of Bob Rimmer, and the two enjoyed a long-standing friendship. Maslow, along with Dr. Rollo May, Dr. Carl Rogers, Drs. Nina and George O'Neil, and many other figures in the human potential movement of the 1970s, was an advocate of loosening the rigidity of monogamous marriage in the interests of supporting greater growth and fulfillment for individuals as well enhancing the depth and quality of marital relationships.

In retrospect, it's difficult to evaluate the success of experiments such as Sandstone and the role of humanistic psychology in changing family forms and sexual mores in America. Tom Hatfield was an enthusiastic participant in the Sandstone experiment until its demise and author of a book documenting the whole project. In a recent personal communication, he confessed that he now questions whether the ideals of synergy and equality were ever achieved. Nevertheless, Sandstone showed many people the power of peak sexual experiences to facilitate personal transformation. The work of best-selling authors such as Alex Comfort (*The Joy of Sex*), Gay Talese (*Thy Neighbor's Wife*), and many other prominent and influential Sandstone guests has deeply penetrated Western culture.

At the same time, the sexual revolution of the 1970s left in its wake the widespread belief that open marriage doesn't work. Open marriage has been lampooned by journalists such as Cyra McFadden, whose satirical writings on Marin County–style human potential marriages in the 1970s[11] are both humorous and on the mark. More recently, the CBS series *Swingtown* has highlighted the escapades of several couples in open marriages in the 1970s and humorously portrays the often messy and dramatic lifestyle of these forerunners of modern polyamory. While the necessary research to conclusively answer the question of whether monogamous marriage "works" any better than open marriage or group marriage has never been done, the data we have indicate that there's no significant difference. I strongly intuit that each works some of the time for some people, with no one option being better than any of the others when it's a good fit for the people involved. We'll explore this topic more thoroughly in future chapters.

THE LAST GENERATION

Dr. James Ramey was another first-wave proponent of alternatives to monogamy whose work is still amazingly contemporary. Jim sought me out in the mid-1980s, and his generous encouragement, advice, and networking until his death in 1995 helped build today's polyamory movement. His book *Intimate Friendships*[12] is still an important resource for researchers and therapists alike, and he and his wife Betty participated in the Kirkridge Conferences described previously. Jim once told me that he'd been involved in intimate friendships, as he preferred to call consensual extramarital relationships, since 1953 and that his research had turned up three line marriages,* one of which had been around since 1815.

Jim first discovered an intimate network in 1952 in Houston, Texas, long before the sexual revolution made such social experiments fashionable and allowed them to become visible to the general public. Unlike many other pioneers of twentieth-century polyamory who came from either academic or religious backgrounds, Jim's career as a self-employed business consultant and his brilliant and original mind gave him the freedom and means to pursue this line of research at a time when such endeavors were risky for those dependent on institutional support. Jim's forty years of research and writing on the topic of alternatives to monogamy and the nuclear family, including two unpublished novels, is an invaluable legacy.

KERISTA VILLAGE

The late twentieth-century Kerista commune, based in San Francisco, California, seems to have been profoundly influenced by Oneida, although the Keristans, as they called themselves, were more inclined to trace their lineage to the Israeli kibbutz movement. However, they were well known for creating the "balanced rotational sleeping schedule," which was designed to prevent pair bonding, and for encounter style "Gestaltorama" groups, which paralleled Oneida's intense group process. They used vasectomies rather than nonejaculation to prevent unplanned pregnancies, held all property in common, and created their own religion that preached *polyfidelity* (another term they invented) as a pathway to worldwide utopia.

Kerista started out in San Francisco's Haight-Ashbury in the aftermath of the Summer of Love as a triad comprised of ex–New Yorkers. The vision held by Brother Jud began to materialize when he was joined by two talented and dynamic young women who adopted the names Even Eve and Blue Jay Way, or Way for short. Eventually, this urban tribe grew to thirty members in three different group marriages, or *best friend identity clusters*

---

*A line marriage is a form of group marriage that appears frequently in Robert Heinlein's novels and in one of Robert Rimmer's as well. In this form of group marriage, new partners who are a generation younger are added periodically, keeping the marriage "alive" and stewarding its assets indefinitely.

(BFICs), and lasted for about twenty years. While the rules of polyfi-delitous engagement prohibited sexual contact of any kind outside of the BFIC, membership status in the BFICs could change almost overnight.

Kerista was perhaps the most visible, the most colorful and long-lived of the many communal experiments that grew out of the sexual revolution of the 1970s. It was also the most rigid and inflexible to the best of my knowledge and rapidly fell apart on Jud's departure. I visited their San Francisco house several times and stayed in contact with some of them after the commune disbanded in 1991. Like the Oneidans before them, many former Keristans opted for monogamy, although some chose to con-tinue in smaller group marriages.

Way once told me, "I paid my dues! If anyone is entitled to monogamy, it's me!" Rather than seeing the choice of monogamy as an indictment of polyfidelity, which was an admittedly challenging practice, especially in the early days, I view this newfound interest in monogamy as natural curiosity on the part of people who had known nothing but polyfidelity as young adults and wanted to explore another way to love.

STAN DALE AND THE HUMAN AWARENESS INSTITUTE

No history of American polyamory would be complete without mention of Stan Dale, who founded the Human Awareness Institute (HAI) in 1968 after a successful career as a radio personality. Like Bob Rimmer, Stan had experienced another approach to sex, love, and intimacy while serving overseas in the military, but in Stan's case, he was exposed to the traditional geisha practices of Japan. I first met Stan in the early 1980s at the northern California home that he and his long time wife Helen shared with Helen's mother until the latter's death. At the time, Stan's other wife Janet had her own home in a nearby city. Stan and Helen were part of the extended family of another group marriage. This group consisted of a core group of four people who'd been living together for about fifteen years at the time, and I was also part of this extended family, which included maybe two dozen people. Every year, there would be a family "reunion" where the entire extended family was invited to gather for all or part of a month devoted to connecting with each other.

Both Stan and I were profoundly influenced by this remarkable group, who'd created the most synergistic relationship of any size I've ever had the privilege to get close to. Much of what I know about love, intimacy, and polyamory I learned from them. And as a result of their contact with Stan, his Sex Workshop evolved into the Love, Sex, and Intimacy Workshops that have now been experienced by over 75,000 people in five different countries. Stan's trainees have carried on his work since his death in 2007. Because Stan was so open about his own triadic marriage and because of our mentors' influence, HAI has always been a space where monogamy and heterosexuality are accepted and respected but not imposed on those who have other preferences.

Shortly after meeting Stan and Helen for the first time, I got a phone call from the producer of the *Phil Donahue Show* who was looking for a guest expert, preferably one with a PhD after her name, to appear on the show with Stan, Helen, and Janet Dale. I said "yes," and it was the outpouring of heartfelt letters I received from those who viewed the show on television that led me to form IntiNet in 1984. At the time, it was the only national organization for responsibly nonmonogamous people—or so I thought. I had no idea when I chose the name IntiNet that *Internet* was soon to become one of the most used words in any language. Nor did I have any idea that about 1,000 miles north of my home in the San Francisco Bay Area, in Eugene, Oregon, Ryam Nearing was starting Polyfidelitous Educational Productions (PEP).

RYAM NEARING AND LOVING MORE MAGAZINE

Ryam Nearing, who founded *Loving More* magazine with me in 1995, was a close friend of the Kerista Villagers, as they sometimes called themselves. Together with her two husbands, Barry and Alan, they formed a polyfidelitous triad who played a key role in the emergence of modern polyfidelity.

Ryam and Barry were all-American high school sweethearts who decided to add Alan to their marriage instead of subtracting Barry. In the 1980s, prior to the explosion of the World Wide Web and before most people had home computers, networking was much slower than it is now. I didn't know that Ryam Nearing and PEP existed until Ryam and I met on the set of the Playboy Channel's *Women on Sex* television program in Hollywood, where we were both being interviewed.

Ryam was recovering from a brush with cancer and had not yet written her book *The Polyfidelity Primer* (1992) and was producing a newsletter and a small conference called PEPCON in the Pacific Northwest. When she decided to move the conference to the University of California at Berkeley, the growth curve accelerated. By the following year, I was organizing the program with her and convinced her to switch to a residential conference at Harbin Hot Springs that quickly doubled the attendance. During this period, there was a brief flirtation between Ryam and her husbands at the time and me and my husband at the time. We were geographically challenged—they were living in Hawaii by this time—and, perhaps more important, the chemistry wasn't there.

Ryam and I worked hard and long for a couple of years to create *Loving More* magazine and expand the Loving More Conferences. She is a woman of great clarity, tolerance, and integrity and was delightful to collaborate with. These were exciting times, filled with television appearances with both our families and radio interviews. Ryam helped provide a sensible, down-to-earth, and reasonable voice for the polyamory movement, which was crucial in those formative days. She was well aware of the importance of creating stable and functional polyamorous relationships if polyamory was to fulfill its promise. In her words, "In entering a love relationship, there's really no free lunch; no way to open your heart and not be vulnerable; no way to take on the karmic bonding of your soul with another's and not accept large responsibilities as part of the deal. Yet this is exactly what I see people expressly looking for—love at no cost, no effort and with no strings. Instead, ecstatic connection and soul union for no money down, no interest charges, and no payments ever. Everybody has been trained to look at financial propositions that promise the impossible with the attitude that 'If it sounds too good to be true, then it is.' Unfortunately in the relationship arena people lose their common sense. . . . Our hearts don't need endless brief encounters or to always move on from one person to another to another looking for some perfect match that won't be so much trouble. Relationships are more than recreation for tonight, and deserve more respect and intention from day one onward. The whole point of loving more for me has always been the increased connection, the amped up intimacy, and the building of a bigger and stronger relationship web. To learn healthy ways to move together through the dances of life amidst a cast of characters growing ever richer in shared experiences."[13]

Despite the tantalizing possibility of taking the magazine mainstream, I eventually began to see that the dream of increasing circulation to a sustainable level that would allow us to hire assistants and maybe take a vacation once in a blue moon was not likely to be realized anytime soon. We both had husbands who were supporting us financially and could afford to work full-time for next to nothing, but I also had a small child and was getting burned out.

In 1993, I introduced Ryam to Brett, who soon became her third and eventually only husband at the Kirkridge Conference. Slowly, our business partnership was replaced by their full-on partnership, and when she became pregnant with his child, I knew this was going to have a major impact on all our lives. I decided it was time for me to move on and leave *Loving More* to them.

GAY, LESBIAN, BISEXUAL, TRANSGENDERED, AND QUEER POLY ACTIVISTS

While the "mainstream" polyamory community has a decidedly heterosexual focus, it's important to recognize that all sexual minorities have played an important role in the spread of polyamorous concepts. Bisexual women in particular have been among the earliest polyamory activists[14] and continue to maintain a high profile in the poly community. The "hot bi babe" continues to be much sought after by polyamorous heterosexual men hoping for a female–female–male triad, and more than half of women in committed polyamorous triads are bisexual. Bisexual men are more cautious about coming out in the polyamorous community (whether as a result of AIDS phobia or homophobia I can't say), and while lesbians and gay men are welcomed in theory, few seem to participate. Celeste West, author of *Lesbian Polyfidelity*, was among the first lesbians to take a stand for polyamory within the lesbian community in the early 1990s, and while many lesbians still prefer monogamy, awareness of polyamory as a legitimate option seems well established.

According to Robin Bauer, a gay female-to-male transsexual who co produced the first international academic conference on polyamory in Germany in 2005, gay men have been practicing nonmonogamy from the get-go and consider heterosexuals to be Johnny-come-latelies. Nevertheless, when gay men attempt more structured multipartner relationships, such as a live-in triad, they seem to have just as much difficulty as hetero- or bisexuals. Polyamory does seem to attract a disproportionate number of transsexuals considering that their numbers are small in the general population. More recently, those who prefer the queer identity as a way of making a statement that they don't fit neatly into any established sexual or gender category have also gravitated toward polyamory.

My impression is that people who have already abandoned heterosexual norms are more likely to question the monogamous norm as well, and surveys have shown that nonmonogamy is common among gay men and, while less common among lesbians, still more frequent than in the heterosexual population. In the early 1990s, when I heard gay theologian and founder of the School of Erotic Massage Joseph Kramer discussing sexual friendship as a survival strategy for gay men in the age of AIDS, a lightbulb lit up in my brain. Kramer was encouraging gay men without primary partners to consider playing erotically with men they already knew and trusted instead of taking risks with strangers or shutting down their sexuality altogether. The concept of friendship, rather than marriage or romance, as a basis for loving, nonmonogamous intimacy that could last a lifetime and enhance health and well-being seemed applicable to man/woman relationships as well as same-gender ones, and I've since found that this idea resonates with many people in the world of polyamory. More committed than a casual fuck buddy or friend with benefits but less all-consuming than a full-on partner, these relationships may represent the future of polyamory. A fuller exploration of sexual friendship is beyond the scope of this book, but I certainly owe a debt of gratitude to Joseph for bringing this concept forward.

BRAD BLANTON AND RADICAL HONESTY

I first became aware of Dr. Brad Blanton when three different intimate friends of mine got excited about his book *Radical Honesty*.[15] One of them invited Brad to offer his ten-day seminar in the San Francisco Bay Area where we lived, and another invited me to Brad's Thought Leaders Conference many years later where I connected with many old and new friends and found one of the most loving and supportive poly-friendly communities I'd yet come across.

Like myself, Brad chose to use his training in clinical psychology to support social change, but his mission has been to support people in telling the truth and creating a culture where lying is not the norm. Truth and love are much more closely related than most people realize, and not just because most of us are in the habit of lying about our sexual attractions. Have you ever noticed that whenever someone honestly expresses what they are feeling, with no blame, defensiveness, self-deception, or hidden agenda, you feel a surge of love? Even if what's been said is not what you wanted to hear, the very act of vulnerable self-disclosure tends to create more intimacy.

While Dr. Blanton is neither for nor against nonmonogamy, he's totally honest about his own polyamorous forays. His work has been enthusiastically embraced by many polyamorous people who recognize that since most of us have been trained to lie to ourselves and to others since birth, we need to learn how to tell the truth, especially when it comes to the sensitive area of sexual attractions and behavior.

Partly as a result of efforts by Dr. Blanton, myself, and other concerned professionals, some psychotherapists are starting to take a more realistic view of monogamy and become less judgmental about other options. As we discussed in the previous chapter, humans are not naturally monogamous, nor are we naturally polyamorous. If we are not honest with ourselves about our sexual desires, our jealousies, and our childish desire to have what we want when we want it, we're not likely to find a way to negotiate this challenging territory harmoniously, with or without committed partner(s).

One step in this direction is to realize that the cultural programming that dictates that mating couples pair up and isolate themselves from others is a relatively recent invention. In the next chapter, we look at evidence from many different disciplines that suggests that bonding and family structures are not limited to dyads.

4

THE ETHICS OF POLYAMORY

In many ways, basic ethical principles remain the same whether or not a relationship is monogamous. For example, honoring one's partner by keeping whatever commitments you have made holds true regardless of the specific content of the commitment. But monogamous relationships are often more resilient when it comes to mistakes and ethical lapses than polyamorous ones. This is partly because polyamorous relationships are inherently more complex and partly because most people lack experience and models for relating in these new ways.

Those of us who were raised in a family where monogamy was the norm have a lifetime of conditioning as a guide. We know what's expected of us. We know what to expect from a partner. We know when something is not as it should be. Consequently, if we find ourselves in a monogamous couple, our relationships may be able to survive on autopilot for a time without any major misunderstandings.

The situation is different for people choosing polyamory. Even if they already know others who are polyamorous, there are many different possibilities for how to structure a polyamorous relationship. In order to stay in integrity, everyone needs to consciously agree on how they will interact (or at least agree to disagree) and then keep the agreements they've made unless they are renegotiated with everyone concerned. Alternatively, if partners decide that their only rule is to behave in accordance with shared

values, the need for integrity and self-awareness becomes even more crucial.

Polyamory by its very nature constitutes a challenge to our age-old
conditioning and frequently stirs up some discomfort. When these inevitable growing pains are intertwined with indignation arising from broken
agreements or insensitive treatment by a thoughtless partner, it becomes
much more difficult to trust the process and surrender to the valuable lessons polyamory can offer. The temptation to throw in the towel and try to
return to what feels safe and familiar while blaming polyamory for one's
suffering can be overwhelming.

Many people, whether they see themselves as monogamous or polyamorous, mistake their partner's lack of empathy, blind spots, or unskilled
communication for an intention to be hurtful. We humans have a tendency to take it personally when another is simply acting out of ignorance
or internal confusion, and this is especially likely when venturing into the
unfamiliar territory of polyamorous relating. While I have seen people,
consciously or unconsciously, using nonmonogamy as a weapon in a battle
with a partner, this is not usually the case. Our legal system takes the position that ignorance is no excuse for breaking the law, but when it comes
to intimate relationships, intentions *do* matter. Perhaps we could say that
good intentions are necessary but not sufficient for ethical polyamory.

Those who wish to establish polyamory as a viable option for intimate
relating would do well to begin by making it a priority to strive to be ethi-
cally impeccable. Ethical behavior starts with the intention to do what is
right and then having the integrity and commitment to carry out that intention. This association between ethics, integrity, and commitment applies
to any type of relationship imaginable, but some of the specifics of what is
considered right or wrong will vary according to whether the relationship
is monogamous and whether the relationship is grounded in the old or
new paradigm. In order to get clear on what constitutes right behavior in a
polyamorous relationship, we must first address the more general question
of the morality of polyamory.

IS POLYAMORY IMMORAL?

As we discussed in chapter 1, polyamory doesn't necessarily involve more
than one partner, but because it allows for this possibility, it is often regarded with suspicion. As we enter the twenty-first century, social norms

and values, particularly those regarding love, sex, and marriage, are still undergoing rapid transformation worldwide. Not only are we in transition, but in today's global village many different cultures and religions with different customs and different perspectives on sexual morality may find themselves at odds. Any valid discussion of morality in the realm of intimacy must address differing values over the centuries and also in different religious or spiritual groups.

In the Western world, many people believe that the Old Testament injunction against adultery automatically makes polyamory morally unacceptable because this assumption went unchallenged for centuries in the wake of the Inquisition and subsequent wave of witch burnings. Yet everyone knows that many of the biblical patriarchs had multiple wives and/or concubines. Father Abraham, warrior-poet King David, and wise King Solomon were all nonmonogamous. Were they committing adultery? Not at all according to anthropologist Helen Fisher, author of *Anatomy of Love* who asserts that in Mosaic law, only intercourse with a married woman was banned. The original intent of the commandment against adultery was to protect the property rights of men to their women, not to prohibit men or even unmarried women from having multiple partners. This is essentially the case with Islamic teachings as well, which allow men to have up to four wives but require women to be monogamous.

In our modern world, people are as likely to question the morality of differential privileges for men and women as they are to accept the morality of age-old patriarchal traditions. *Morality* is sometimes viewed as a synonym for *sexual sobriety*, and commitment and fidelity are often assumed to imply exclusivity. It's important to acknowledge that moral parameters involve judgments about what constitutes right behavior in many domains, not just sex.

In many ways, the gap between values held in old- and new-paradigm relationships is far greater than the gap in values between monogamy and patriarchal polygamy. Let's review the ethical guidelines for old- and new-paradigm relating before going on to explore the perspectives of some contemporary religious and spiritual leaders and their teachings relevant to monogamous and nonmonogamous unions.

OLD- AND NEW-PARADIGM VALUES

Many observers have commented that our culture is in the midst of a paradigm shift in the realms of love, family, gender roles, sexuality, and relationship in general. Futurist FM Esfandiary[1] often emphasized that the closer to home a paradigm shift is, the more we tend to resist it. People feel more threatened by a change in our understanding of love than a change in the way physicists understand atomic particles. Writing in the early 1980s, Esfandiary described the process as follows:

"In today's world, virtually all areas of our society are undergoing vast upheavals; the trend, especially in organizations, corporations, and businesses, is toward despecialization, decentralization, denationalization, and diversification. In the face of such significant change, it is crazy to think that the home will remain intact and somehow miraculously unchanged. Our homes, our social life and our interpersonal connections are undergoing precisely the same kind of evolution. In the 1950s, 75–80 percent of families in the U.S. were traditional (breadwinner husband, homemaker wife, two or more kids); today, that figure is less than 7 percent."[2]

In the old paradigm, the stability and longevity of a relationship are its most valued attributes. Dependency, both financial and emotional, serves the function of keeping spouses together and is not seen as a problem. As the twenty-first century dawns, stability is still valued by many, but dependency is more likely to be recognized as an impediment to deep intimacy and a source of conflict and dissatisfaction than a positive or necessary condition for a stable marriage. Nevertheless, the old-paradigm emphasis on maintaining the status quo is still strongly held.

In the new paradigm, the presence of acceptance and unconditional love tends to take precedence over everything else. What this means in practice is that allowing the form of the relationship to shift—for example, from romance to friendship or from a closed marriage to an open marriage or marriage to divorce while maintaining positive regard, caring, and support for all those involved—is the primary ethical standard in the new paradigm. Staying married while quietly hating each other and remaining stuck in destructive patterns would not be seen as desirable in the new paradigm but could be perfectly acceptable in the old paradigm.

Some people seem to interpret the new paradigm's appreciation for impermanence as permission to duck out the back door when fear, conflicts, or what seems to be a more desirable partner come along. Allowing avoidance, cowardice, and opportunism to determine one's actions is no more ethical in the new paradigm than in the old. With the freedom to ask that relationships be allowed to shift comes the responsibility to listen to your inner voice for guidance as to what constitutes loyalty and commitment, which are no less important in the new paradigm than in the old even though their focus may broaden.

In the old paradigm, loyalty and commitment to spouse and blood family are an important moral code. In the new paradigm, the sphere of commitment sometimes expands to include all of life. FM Esfandiary expresses it this way:

> The single individual who is relatively free of imprinting can function with versatility, freedom and autonomy, and can begin to express a new kind of commitment—commitment not to a specific individual, not to an attachment figure, but to a much greater environment. If it is possible for us to identify with and be committed to a specific person or group, it ought to become possible for us to reprogram so that we can begin to *identify with and be committed to ALL HUMANITY!* If we can transcend imprinting, it is possible to empathize with *everybody* . . . Individuals who are committed to their creative work, to causes, jobs and movements, are already moving in this direction of greater commitment. Ultimately, commitment to planet and all humanity will replace commitment to clan, family, or nation.[3]

Another important value difference between old and new paradigms is in the area of disclosure. In the old paradigm, with its emphasis on stability, it's considered appropriate to keep secrets, withhold information, or say things one knows to be false if speaking the truth might rock the boat. The norm for the upper classes in much of Europe and parts of the United States has long been to tolerate extramarital affairs as long as they are kept discrete and don't interfere with family obligations.[4] In the new paradigm, a higher value is placed on being totally honest or transparent toward the goal of creating more authentic and growth-producing relationships. In the old paradigm, controlling your partner's behavior, by lying about your own actions if necessary, is valued over telling the truth and accepting the consequences.

Riane Eisler has written extensively about the paradigm shift in attitudes toward love, sex, and the family, which she characterizes as a shift from domination of the feminine by the masculine to partnership and equality between men and women.[5] In the old dominator paradigm, pain and fear of punishment are the primary motivators, she says. In the new paradigm of partnership, pleasure is a core value. Those actions that contribute to shared pleasure are considered right and good. Violence and coercion are not condoned for any reason and are especially anathema when used to subjugate others.

In my 2005 book *The Seven Natural Laws of Love*,[6] I discuss the nature of love in the new paradigm at length. The brief summary of the differences between the old and new paradigms for love mentioned previously merely highlights the major differences in values and beliefs. Now let's see what some contemporary religious leaders have to say about the ethics of polyamory.

CONTEMPORARY CHRISTIAN VIEWPOINTS

In chapter 2, we discussed the important role that progressive Christian clergy have played in challenging the monogamous standard since the nineteenth century. Twenty-first century Episcopalian theologian Carter Heyward[7] takes a more neutral stance by emphasizing the familiar old-paradigm value of fidelity or faithfulness while giving it a new-paradigm twist. Her interpretation of faith involves "trusting that each of us is being honest with the other; that each knows and cares about the other on the basis of who [they] really are, rather than on the basis of who we might wish [them] to be; and that each desires the other's well-being." In other words, she is emphasizing unconditional love and honesty rather than form as the foundation for the ethics of intimacy.

Dr. Heyward asserts that fidelity does not require monogamy, but it does require that we be honest with each other and honor each other's feelings. In her view, any sexual option, including monogamy, can be chosen in alienation or in fidelity. Heyward warns that monogamy can easily be used to shield spouses from their real feelings, fears, and yearnings and so prevent growth in a relationship. An "unexamined, static commitment to monogamy" can just as easily be used to destroy fidelity as to preserve it, insists Heyward.

In Dr. Heyward's contemporary Christian viewpoint, both polyamory and monogamy are morally neutral. Morality is a matter of how we conduct ourselves within our chosen lifestyle rather than adhering to any particular form. She believes that while historically monogamy benefited women and children by providing some measure of economic security by obligating men to provide for their families and also served to protect women from unwanted sexual advances from other men, it is no longer necessary. Today's women have achieved sufficient equality to provide for themselves. Both monogamy and polyamory are moral options if chosen with the intent of building and sustaining trust in a relationship where extraordinary love is present, according to Heyward.

At the height of the sexual revolution, Dr. Robert Francoeur, a married Catholic priest, proposed the concept of "flexible monogamy," in which sexual relationships with partners other than one's spouse could be permitted within the context of a lifelong marriage. A similar concept was proposed by Christian laymen Rustum and Della Roy in their 1968 book *Honest Sex*[8] and later popularized by George and Nena O'Neill as *Open Marriage*.[9]

Dr. Francoeur's position is that a long-lasting marriage that allows for outside sexual partners is more stable and better suited to the pressures of modern life than a series of short-lived monogamous marriages. Thus far, what little data we have suggest that there's no difference in longevity between open marriage and closed marriage, but I strongly intuit that overall monogamy is not a significant variable in predicting longevity. Nevertheless, Dr. Francoeur is clearly placing a higher moral value on stability and longevity than on sexual exclusivity. In other words, he is suggesting that the moral litmus test for relationship ethics be "does it preserve the relationship or destroy the relationship?" This is an interesting blending of paradigms that marries the old-paradigm value of longevity to the new-paradigm acceptance of allowing greater flexibility of form while continuing to give greater weight to longevity.

CONTEMPORARY JUDAISM

Rabbi Arthur Waskow, a respected leader in the movement for Jewish Renewal, points out that while the asserted norm for most modern Jews is sexual monogamy, the norm is often disobeyed in practice because it's untenable for many couples. His recommendation is that couples make their own decisions about whether to be monogamous and that sexual relations outside of marriage be considered adultery only if one of the partners betrays a commitment to monogamy.[10]

Dr. Waskow also suggests that in some circumstances, the decision to engage in extramarital sex may be the most caring and loving course of action. He gives the example of a man whose wife had been institutionalized for a number of years with an incurable and debilitating illness. The man was very devoted in his emotional and financial support of his wife, but he was also lonely. Years passed, and he became involved with another woman. He didn't want to divorce his wife, but he wanted to include his new partner into his life as completely as possible. Rabbi Waskow's view is that the man was operating in full integrity and should be supported by his religious community. He believes that "the new sexual ethics emerge not from a commander outside and above us, but from the need to make worthy, honest, decent, and stable loving connections among ourselves."

Dr. Waskow reminds us that up until 1,000 years ago, Western Jews could legitimately have more than one wife, and the same was true for Eastern Jews up to the late twentieth century. This practice was abandoned partly for the protection of women and partly because of the judgments of Christians who found polyamory to be one more excuse for anti-Semitism. Perhaps it would be preferable, he asserts, to end the prohibition against nonmonogamy and allow both men and women to take more than one mate. The question, he concludes, is one of whether de facto adultery is less dangerous than de jure polyamory.

Rabbi Gershon Winkler, author of *Sacred Secrets: The Sanctity of Sex in Jewish Law and Lore*,[11] also cites the old Jewish practice of *pilagshut*, which literally means "half marriage." Similar to the pagan custom of *handfasting* or today's *domestic partners*, this was a legitimate alternative to marriage for thousands of years that allowed men and women to declare themselves partners, live together, and have children if they wished with no social stigma. Neither government nor religious institutions were involved, and the *pilagshut* could also be dissolved at will. Because it was not technically marriage, women as well as men could have more than one *pilagshut* without committing adultery as long as they refrained from institutionalized marriage.

Ancient commentaries on *pilagshut* address its wholesome and beneficial use while condemning circumstances in which it might be detrimental to those involved. Winkler cites many rabbinical sources and sacred texts blessing nonmarital sex and concludes that while some rabbis condemned the practice, they are in the minority. Traditional Jewish law regarding sex is not what most people today assume it to be, he concluded.

EASTERN RELIGIONS

Hinduism, like Judeo-Christian theology, finds itself facing the paradox of advocating monogamy as an ethical standard while immensely popular

mythologies, such as the *Mahabharata*, feature wives with multiple husbands. Lord Krishna, one of the most beloved of all Hindu figures, is said
to have had 16,008 wives. In ancient India, multiple wives were permitted
depending on one's caste and ability to support them, and it was not until
1955 that the Hindu Marriage Act made polygamy illegal.[12] Prior to this,
Hindu law sanctioned polygamy if it served to strengthen the family but
not for purely hedonist purposes.

Hindu spiritual teachers tend to look on the family as the major source of
attachment and karmic entanglements and so favor celibacy or monogamy
or, in the case of Osho, also recognize the merit of being single and polyamorous as an option[13] for dedicated spiritual seekers. Some might challenge categorizing Osho as a Hindu teacher despite his Hindu upbringing,
but the elaborate sculptures of multipartner sexual activity adorning the
walls at the ancient Tantric temples at Khajuraho and elsewhere suggest
that Hinduism has a long history of recognizing the spiritual significance
of eroticism, both metaphorically and otherwise.[14]

While traveling in India, I visited the abandoned palace of the sixteenth-
century Muslim emperor Akbar at Fatehpur Sikri in Uttar Pradesh. Within
the palace grounds is the tomb of the Sufi saint Salim Chisti of the Chisti
Order, which is known for its emphasis on love, tolerance, and openness.
Chisti was the revered teacher and close adviser of Emperor Akbar. I
learned that Akbar had three wives, one Muslim, one Hindu, and one
Christian, and that each had her own wing in the palace artistically designed in the style of her own faith. I loved the creative use of polygamy to
make this typically Chisti ecumenical statement.

The nineteenth-century mystic Baha'u'llah, founder of the Baha'i
faith, was a product of the Muslim culture, which continues to permit
men to have more than one wife. As a staunch advocate of the rights
of women and the importance of the family, Baha'u'llah had concerns
about the ethics of multiple marriages. His position was that in an ethical and moral marriage, each spouse must be treated exactly equally. He
condemned polygamous marriage on the grounds that this condition was
rarely met. In so doing, he became perhaps the first Islamic spokesper-
son to articulate modern polyamorous ethics. More mainstream Muslims
defend the practice of polyamory by pointing out that the second wife
and her children have greater protection under the law than the unmarried mistress of a married man.[15]

Buddhist doctrine, or dharma, focuses on the effects of our sexual
acts rather than the acts themselves. The dharma teaches that those acts

that cause pain and harm to others or disturbance in ourselves should be avoided. According the ancient *Six Paramitas of the Bodhisattva*, a moral person having sex with another must consider his or her own happiness, that of his or her companion, and that of the third person who will be most affected by the situation. If these three people are not harmed, then polyamory is not adultery and meets Buddhist ethical standards.[16] Classical Buddhist teachings show no general preference for one form of relationship over another, except in the case of monks, who are required to avoid attachments. Instead, Buddhism considers what is most appropriate for particular people in particular places at particular times.

Contemporary Buddhist teachers in the West from a variety of schools, including high-profile individuals such as the Dalai Lama and Thich Nhat Hanh, tend to promote monogamy as a Buddhist ethical standard despite the absence of dharmic support and despite the acceptance of nonmonogamy in many predominantly Buddhist countries. Perhaps, like the Jews in Western Europe during medieval times, they are trying to adapt Buddhism to fit Christian society and make it more palatable to westerners.

East–West psychology professor Jorge Ferrer suggests that the celibacy vows taken by Buddhist monks limit their direct experience of these matters and encourages Buddhists to go straight to the source, pointing out that the Buddha himself advocated polyamory over monogamy in certain situations. He relates a story told in the *Jataka 200* of a Brahmin who asks the Buddha for advice on choosing husbands for his four daughters. The Brahmin says, "One was fine and handsome, one was old and well advanced in years, the third a man of family [noble birth], and the fourth was good." "Even though there be beauty and the like qualities," the Buddha answered, "a man is to be despised if he fails in virtue. Therefore the former is not the measure of a man; those that I like are the virtuous." After hearing this, the Brahmin gave *all* his daughters to the virtuous suitor.[17]

Ferrer concludes that from the Buddhist perspective of skillful means (*upaya*), the key factor in evaluating the appropriateness of any intimate connection may not be its form but rather its power to eradicate the suffering of self and others. He also favors the nondogmatic and pragmatic approach of historical Buddhism, which, like historical Hinduism, was not attached to any specific relationship structure but was essentially guided by a radical emphasis on liberation. These ethical criteria are found in many contemporary teachings as well from humanistic psychology to *The Work* of Byron Katie.

NONDENOMINATIONAL SPIRITUALITY AND HUMANISM

Byron Katie stands out among contemporary spiritual teachers in many ways. An ordinary California housewife who spontaneously awakened in the midst of a personal crisis, she is not beholden to any traditional lineage, and her teachings are completely content and culture free, similarly to the Advaita of the venerated Indian sage Ramana Maharshi. Arguing with reality is a lost cause, Katie tells us. Instead, questioning our thoughts while taking actions that support ourselves and those we care for is her prescription for a happy and ethical life.[18] She is one of the few spiritual leaders who is willing to openly discuss her own reasons for choosing monogamy while refraining from advocating one form of relationship over another.[19]

Dr. Carl Rogers is one of the most respected and influential of all the gifted therapists to emerge from the humanistic psychology movement. In the early 1970s, Rogers predicted that the "attitude of possessiveness" in marriage would be greatly diminished by the twenty-first century.[20] Like many of his humanistic colleagues, Rogers refused to make judgments about people's lifestyle choices and instead sought to understand and evaluate their experience according to whether it was growth producing for all involved or, in the case of couples, whether it deepened their connection and enhanced the quality of their relationship.

Nobel Laureate Bertrand Russell is perhaps the most illustrious of a long line of philosophers and ethicists who have argued that sexual morality is too important to the happiness and well-being of us all to be determined by tribal traditions, superstition, politics, economics, and religious taboos. The famous mathematician urges that logic and rational thought be applied to determining what sexual ethics are appropriate in modern life while citing functional examples from other cultures to expand the universe of possibilities.[21]

Writing in the early twentieth century, Russell accepted premarital and extramarital sex on the grounds that they contributed to love, happiness in marriage, and great art, creating a storm of controversy. Today, his analysis offers a framework for a new sexual ethic.

TOWARD A NEW SEXUAL ETHIC

The contemporary religious and spiritual perspectives summarized here suggest that in evaluating the morality of any lovestyle, it is less important to blindly follow a particular rule or custom than it is to ask the following:

Does this relationship have a positive effect on those who are in it, on any children produced by it, and on the rest of the world?
Does this relationship effectively serve the basic functions of family life?
Does this relationship support the continued evolution of humanity, the plant and animal kingdoms, and the planet?

After considering the accumulated wisdom of today's twenty-first-century global village, I suggest the following values as a basis for a new sexual ethic. In addressing each one, examples are given of how it would apply in a polyamorous relationship.

Honesty

It's hard to trust a person who lies, deceives, or withholds information unless we are speaking about trusting that someone may not be telling the truth. Being scrupulously honest with yourself and your partners is especially important in polyamory because honest communication is the best way of handling the fears and jealousies that inevitably arise from time to time. Trust can then be based on the certain knowledge that your partners are giving you their unedited truth about their feelings and behavior. This gives your relationships the secure grounding they need to remain comfortable when exploring polyamory and allows you to distinguish imagined threats from reality.

Hiding your polyamorous nature from prospective partners who may reject you out of hand may be tempting, but it is not honest. In the long run, it will backfire. Honesty includes being clear with your partners about your intentions and priorities. Of course, you must use good judgment about when to disclose something that may be difficult for your partners to hear, but letting fears about hurting someone's feelings serve as an excuse for keeping secrets is not ethical. Withholding your true thoughts and feelings does just as much damage to you as to your partners by replacing intimacy with alienation and blocking the free flow of loving energy. Sooner or later, you will find that the emotional withdrawal and resentment that invariably follow from not speaking your truth are deadening your love and your sexual response. Sustainable intimacy requires total honesty.

Nonmonogamy is often associated with scandals such as the revelations that conservative South Carolina Governor Mark Sanford used private and state planes to secretly visit his mistress in Argentina in 2009.[22] Newspapers made the most of reports that Sanford told his staff he was hiking the Appalachian Trail to cover up his trip to Argentina to see his "soul mate." Meanwhile, Sanford's wife and four sons moved out of the governor's mansion and were said to be struggling to reconcile. Some Republicans called for impeachment and said that Sanford had brought "extreme dishonor and shame" on the state, but Sanford's lawyer said he believed that the governor would be exonerated. Too many people still think of cases like this when they hear the word *polyamory*, and only consistent adherence to a standard of honesty will establish a distinction.

Commitment

The type of commitments made depends on the form a relationship takes and whether you are working from an old- or a new-paradigm model. However, all grounded relationships involve some kind of commitment. Regardless of the specifics, meaningful sex creates a lifelong bond. It is simply not ethical to thoughtlessly discard lovers like yesterday's garbage. In an ongoing polyamorous relationship of any kind, all partners need to know that their beloved will not duck out of the relationship on a whim because they got scared or because they found someone else who wants them to be monogamous. Without a commitment to working to strengthen and enhance existing relationships, adding new partners can result only in jealousy.

If your partner is not satisfied with the quality of your interaction, he or she is probably not going to be happy about someone else getting what he or she wants. Not all relationships can last a lifetime, and there are many good reasons to create some distance, but commitment means making an effort to resolve conflicts. Commitment doesn't have to mean promising to stick around forever no matter what. It does mean having a lifelong intention to support each other in whatever ways seem appropriate. Marking time until someone you like better comes along is not ethical, especially if you don't make it clear that this is what you're doing. The easiest way to avoid this dilemma is not to engage in marginal relationships. Should you find yourself involved with someone who doesn't feel "right" to you, it's best to be honest about your lack of commitment. Give him or her the option to end the relationship if she or he is looking for something deeper. If you have agreements with any of your partners that you will end other sexual relationships at their request, this also needs to be communicated to new partners.

Single people who don't intend to create a primary relationship with anyone can clarify the extent and limitations of the commitment they are willing to make. A single person can let partners know about their commitment to remain single and nonmonogamous from the start so that there is less room for misunderstanding and disappointment later on. Whether or not you intend to remain single, keep in mind that a commitment to something higher than yourself or your partner, whether that be truth, the Divine, higher self, integrity, or whatever you hold sacred, is a good way to anchor a relationship within a larger context.

Agreements and Decision Making

Couples have many areas of life where they need to reach agreements about how they will handle things that impact both of them. However, when it comes to agreeing about whom they will have sex with, it's fairly straightforward in a monogamous relationship: both partners are agreeing to forsake all others. In polyamory, everyone must decide which, when, how, and to what extent multiple partners will be included. There are literally thousands of different agreements that people can make about how they will conduct their intimate relationships. There are also different decision-making processes that can be used by two or more people. It's important to learn about the different options that are possible and to discern which may be appropriate for your situation. Polyamory is a lot like democracy—it works best with educated and involved citizens.

As we enter the twenty-first century, models for successful polyamorous relationships are increasingly visible, but there is no getting around the fact that there is more than one right way to do it, and no one model works for everyone. Self-knowledge is again an essential prerequisite in knowing what kinds of agreements you want. Making agreements you don't think you can live with in order to keep the peace usually doesn't work. It's far better to let your conflicts surface early on than to feel constrained, co-erced, or victimized later on.

Marvin and Sheila are a new couple in their early sixties who have decided to marry after dating for nearly a year. Sheila, who was divorced after twenty-five years of marriage to a possessive and demanding hus-band, is clear that she does not want to make a monogamous commitment. She loves Argentinean Tango and usually goes out dancing several times a week. She wants to share her life with Marvin, and she also wants the freedom to flirt and to explore sexually with other men if the situation pres-ents itself. After Marvin's wife died, he had a relationship with a woman who was in an open marriage for many years. Because of this experience, he's fairly comfortable with Sheila's desires, and he's clear that he doesn't want the distraction and complication of more than one relationship for himself.

In his previous marriage, Marvin had also discovered that he preferred to allow his wife to be the boss. "We were both dominant personalities, and in the beginning we fought about everything all the time. It was pretty unpleasant," he told me. "After a while I decided to try letting her decide if we disagreed on something. To my surprise, I found that I liked being more submissive in our relationship, and she liked this too. We got along very well from then on. I would do this again in any intimate relation-ship."

Marvin came to me for help in drawing up a set of agreements that would be acceptable to both of them. Marvin trusted Sheila's commitment to their relationship and didn't feel the need for sexual exclusivity, but he didn't want his comfortable, predictable, and fairly conventional lifestyle disturbed. He already knew that there were two situations he'd find dif-ficult. He didn't want Sheila to have sex with other men in their shared home, and he didn't want Sheila to get involved with anyone who was part of their social circle. Sheila was fine with these conditions. I asked how he felt about Sheila spending the night elsewhere, which was something he hadn't thought about but quickly decided that this would be okay for him as long as he knew she wasn't coming home.

"Do you want Sheila to phone you at midnight if she suddenly realizes she wants an overnight that wasn't planned on? Or does she have to tell you before she goes out?" I asked. Marvin wasn't sure at first, but after some conversation with Sheila, they found a solution. She would text him to keep him informed of her plans as they evolved.

Marvin was reluctant to meet any of Sheila's potential lovers, something that Sheila wanted. When I pointed out that he might be missing an opportunity to make some new male friends as well as sending a clear message to any suitors that Sheila already had a primary partner, Marvin agreed to try this out and see how he felt about it before rejecting it out of hand. This led to his realizing that he wanted Sheila to agree to tell any prospective lovers that she was already "taken" and to reserve two nights a week for him. Sheila again agreed with these requests and wanted Marvin's okay for occasional vacations with other men. I suggested that they get more specific about how often and how long she might be gone. Marvin's favorite part of their agreement was his promise to Sheila that he would remain monogamous. She was quite willing to offer him reciprocal privileges to see other women, but he was clear that he wasn't interested. He wanted to keep it simple, and he knew he didn't have the sex drive he'd had in his youth. One woman was enough for him. Sheila was quite touched by Marvin's devotion, and he delighted in freely giving her this gift.

With a less mature couple, I might have been skeptical about whether all these agreements could be kept and whether they might create some resentment. However, Marvin and Sheila knew themselves well, and knew what they wanted and what they could deliver. They had overlooked a few potential problem areas but were able to easily reach agreement on how their open relationship would work.

Integrity

Integrity involves doing whatever you've agreed to do, whether it's as mundane as doing the dishes or as central to your relationship as keeping an agreement to practice safe sex with other partners. Without integrity, commitments and agreements are worse than useless. You can make hundreds of agreements and break every single one of them. In fact, the more agreements you make, the more likely it is that some will be broken.

One definition for integrity is wholeness. Some go so far as to say that integrity is a necessary condition for workability.[23] Interestingly enough, wholeness is also the original meaning of health, suggesting that regardless of the form, healthy, workable relationships exist among people with sufficient self-knowledge and self-acceptance to be aware of all the internal parts of themselves. Otherwise, one part is liable to make an agreement that some other part has no intention of keeping. This often happens with people who say they will be monogamous and refuse to admit that they also have a desire for other sexual partners.

People who have recognized and accepted their polyamorous nature may have an easier time staying in integrity because once their polyamorous parts understand that their needs and desires will be honored, these parts may be more amenable to exercising some restraint and finding means of expression that are not harmful to others. There is no guarantee of this, however, and a polyamorous person operating without integrity can wreak havoc.

Integrity in polyamorous relationships also means that a commitment to one partner that involves the cooperation of another partner can be made only by first getting agreement from all concerned. For example, if Joe promises Stephanie that he will attend a family reunion in another state with her next summer and he has a standing agreement with Mary that he won't go out of town with another partner if she has to work overtime and can't pick their children up from the day care center by closing time, Joe may find himself in trouble if he hasn't first cleared this exception with Mary.

Equity

Earlier in this chapter, we addressed the ethics and values of patriarchal polygamy, which allows differential privileges to men and to women. We also briefly touched on the question of decision making and how power is shared between partners. While there are different ways to structure intimate relationships independently of the form these relationships take, if equity is not present in a relationship, it is neither ethical nor sustainable.

Equity means treating others with fairness, and while fairness is always a judgment call, it suggests that all parties have equal power for determining the quality of their lives even though they may have different roles, duties, or responsibilities. Equity is characteristic of what Riane Eisler has called "partnership culture," as contrasted with "dominator culture," in which it is assumed that one gender has the right to control the other gender, with violence if necessary. Where equity is present, one person may still assume more leadership than the other(s), or different people may assume leadership in different arenas or decide to rotate responsibilities, but the process of making decisions is one that is mutually agreed on as beneficial for everyone. This style has sometimes been described as "power with" rather than "power over," or mutually empowering.

Now let's take a look at some relationships that illustrate how the form of the relationship is less important than the previously discussed ethical principles in determining the value and impact of the relationship.

UNHEALTHY MONOGAMY LEADS TO UNHEALTHY POLYAMORY

Vic and Christy had been more or less happily married for twelve years when they met Alice and Jack at a party. Christy is the stay-at-home mom of two young children, and Vic travels extensively for his job. His frequent absences were the biggest stress on their relationship with Christy feeling resentful about being left alone with the children and Vic missing his family while on the road.

Alice and Jack had also been married for nearly twelve years and had two children the same ages as Vic and Christy's. Jack ran his successful computer business from home with administrative support from Alice, so the two were together almost all the time. At the time they met Vic and Christy, Alice was considering divorce because she was fed up with Jack's verbal abuse and feared his explosive temper but was even more afraid of the financial consequences of leaving her husband.

The two couples became increasingly close, and their children became best friends. Christy and the kids often spent time with Alice and her family while Vic was away on business and soon found herself falling in love with Jack. One weekend, Christy suggested that the foursome explore sexually together, and they all enjoyed the experience so much that it soon became a regular part of their interaction. All was well until Vic became aware of the depth of Christy's feelings for Jack and at the same time found that he was reluctant to open his heart more fully to Alice, who clearly preferred Vic to her own husband. Sex with Alice and Jack was fine with Vic, but he felt that love should be reserved for spouses. He valued his family life and his role as a father and didn't want to play with fire. He wanted to break off the relationship with Alice and Jack entirely, but Christy refused and instead suggested that they all consult me.

Christy and Jack had developed a sexual chemistry so strong that it was nearly palpable. Not only was Vic afraid that Christy might leave him for Jack, but he feared that casual friends would suspect that they were having an affair and was angry about their lack of discretion. Christy's reassurances that she had no intention of breaking up their family fell on deaf ears.

For the moment, this quadrangle was meeting all her needs, and she was convinced that if only Vic would stop resisting, everyone would live happily ever after. Initially, I worked just with Christy and Vic to address Vic's jealousy and Christy's old resentments about feeling dominated by Vic. Christy and Vic made rapid progress in resolving these issues, but when Jack and Alice failed to follow through on making an appointment for themselves and when all four were unable to find a time to come in together, I sensed that a happy and healthy foursome was not a likely prospect.

After some months, Alice and Jack decided to seek help with their relationship. Alice was struggling to forgive Jack for his past behavior. She appreciated that he behaved in a more loving and supportive way when Christy was around, but at the same time she was hurt and angry about the verbal abuse he still dished out to her when they were alone. She often vented her frustration privately with Vic, adding fuel to Vic's animosity toward Jack for capturing Christy's heart. Vic's instincts were at least partly correct. He and Christy might not want to swap spouses, but Alice and Jack certainly did. Christy's vision was that of a four-way group marriage, and while it *was* a good match in many ways, Vic's doubts were well founded. Vic and Christy's relationship was reasonably functional, but Alice and Jack's was not. Had they swapped spouses, they almost certainly would have found the same dynamics showing up with their new partners.

This vignette is a good example of unhealthy monogamy leading to unhealthy polyamory. The sex was good, but the emotional chaos became a downward spiral that soon wore everyone out. Christy's vision of including others into one big happy family to create support for herself and her children while Vic was out of town on business was a healthy impulse. With a less dysfunctional couple, it might have worked, but her sexual and romantic attraction to Jack blinded her to the reality that Jack and Alice's marriage was falling apart. For Jack and Alice, polyamory was an avoidance of their issues, not a solution. Soon after the two couples stopped seeing each other, Alice began an affair with a recently divorced single father. She divorced Jack a year later.

HEALTHY MONOGAMY LEADS
TO HEALTHY POLYAMORY

Both Janice and Peter were happily married to their respective spouses when they met at a party for nonmonogamous couples. At first, they thought their attraction was primarily sexual, but gradually the relationship expanded into a full-blown love affair. Peter and his wife Stacy felt very secure in their marriage of ten years, and Stacy was happy to have Peter occupied while she pursued her passion for ice skating. Janice's husband, Ian, was fully engaged in growing his prosperous company and felt strongly about supporting Janice's freedom to love others. With some trepidation, Ian welcomed the challenge of overcoming his own feelings of jealousy and envy. All four were young, attractive, successful professionals who were content with their lives and optimistic about their future. Both couples were committed to their families, had clear agreements about how to handle outside relationships, and placed a high priority on maintaining a satisfying marriage.

As time passed, Janice and Peter found themselves facing difficulties that had never emerged in their harmonious and comfortable marriages. After almost breaking up because of repeated conflicts, they sought me out for help. It soon became apparent to me that Janice and Peter had found in each other a fabulous mirror for their unresolved childhood issues that simply wasn't present with their highly compatible spouses. From the vantage point of marital stability, they were fortunate that the stormy, passionate, and richly productive quality of their interaction had shown up outside their marriages.

I quickly pointed out to Janice and Peter that working out their conflicts was strictly voluntary. Each of them had full and rewarding lives independently of each other. They could simply stop seeing each other and find other growth opportunities that were less challenging and easier to manage. After considering this option, they decided to go for it and use the emotional upheaval that each triggered in the other as a starting point for healing their childhood wounds.

Stacy and Ian had done their best to be supportive of their partners, but both were relieved when Janice and Peter's relationship began to stabilize. Stacy and Ian recognized the value for Janice and Peter of resolving their conflicts but were getting disturbed by the increasing drama that was rippling into their respective marriages. Neither Stacy nor Ian wanted to pull rank and ask their spouses to break off their relationship, though they knew that such a request would be complied with. Once Janice and Peter began taking responsibility for their own healing, Stacy and Ian could happily embrace the situation.

These four people are good examples of people for whom polyamory is a workable choice. Not only did each couple have a highly functional marriage, but each individual had a variety of personality traits and skills that are necessary for polyamorous relating, as we shall see in the next chapter.

5

THE POLYAMOROUS PERSONALITY

Most people never stop to ask themselves whether their personal characteristics make them better suited for monogamy or for polyamory or for each at different stages in life. While many young people growing up today have more awareness than previous generations that they do have options when it comes to their choice of lovestyle, it's still unusual to make a conscious choice whether to practice monogamy. Even more unusual is to come to an understanding that polyamory is not an identity that dictates having multiple partners but rather a fluid process of checking in with oneself to see what feels appropriate with a given person in a given situation. Instead, we tend to be influenced by the conditioning we receive in the families we grow up in or the prevailing social norms. This holds true whether we imitate our parents or vow never to be like them and deliberately do the opposite.

Ann's father had many illicit affairs. Ann's mother suffered silently. When Ann was seven, they divorced with much hostility. Ann was determined to have a solid monogamous marriage with a husband who would never leave her or cheat on her. Jeff's father also had many illicit affairs that his mother pretended not to notice while enjoying a variety of sports and activities at her church. When Jeff was seven, his parents peacefully divorced, and his father soon remarried. Jeff modeled himself on his father and usually had several girlfriends at once but decided to always tell the truth about being nonmonogamous. When he married, he chose a woman who also wanted an open marriage. Cindy's parents were unhappily married for fifty years. They rarely had sex with each other or with anyone else as far as Cindy knew. Cindy tried hard to find a husband but couldn't seem to meet the right man and began to wonder if she was a lesbian. Then she became involved with a bisexual couple and happily settled into an open triad.

While heterosexual monogamous marriage is still the ideal in much of the world, subcultures where polyamory, bisexuality, or homosexuality are the norm are increasingly visible and gaining in respectability. More and more people are deciding to remain single or to live together without getting married, especially if they don't plan to have children. Since the sexual revolution of the 1960s and 1970s, there is a new generation who grew up in nontraditional families where gender roles, sexual orientation, and/or relational orientation were much more fluid than in the past. While the lifestyle choices of these young adults have not yet been studied scientifically, it's my impression that in general they are much more comfortable with themselves and their sexuality. As we will see in chapter 8, many of them still gravitate toward heterosexual and/or monogamous relationships, but they are more willing to experiment with different kinds of relationships and have many of the skills and personality traits that contribute to successful polyamorous relationships.

Some mental health professionals have long held the unfounded opinion that polyamorous people are disturbed in some way, and some try to dissuade clients from practicing polyamory or attribute their relationship problems to their rejection of monogamy. But these judgments often turn out to be a reflection of personal and societal bias. Those practicing polyamory share the same psychological problems as the rest of the population, but a number of studies conducted in the 1980s found no differences in psychological symptoms or quality of relationships between those practicing polyamory and those who were monogamous.[1]

While the polyamorous personality has not been found to be pathological on the whole and while there is much diversity among those classified as polyamorous, many polyamorous people do seem to share certain qualities, and it's my impression that certain personality types are more likely than others to choose polyamory (whether or not they identify as polyamorous). Some of these factors may have as much to do with the personality traits of those willing to make choices that do not conform to social norms as with polyamory itself, but at this time, both variables are generally involved in making polyamorous choices. In addition, the factors predicting compatibility among those in multipartner relationships are somewhat different from those relevant to dyadic relationships. In the absence of research that would address all these questions, this chapter presents a combination of my own clinical and anecdotal observations as well as a synthesis of the ideas of other authors and researchers in the field.

As we've discussed in previous chapters, there are many different styles of polyamorous relationships. Open marriage, intimate networks, and group marriages appeal to different types of people and require different strengths and skills. It's difficult to identify a single individual who represents such a diverse universe, so I will share a few composite pictures.

QUINTESSENTIAL POLYAMOROUS WOMEN

Elaine is thirty-five and has three children, the youngest still in diapers, and works part time as a clothing designer. She's been married to William for ten years, and for the past four years she's also had a close relationship with Timothy. "I almost decided to stop seeing Timothy after Julia was born, but in the end I realized that I receive so much from him, it's worth the extra time and energy. I couldn't do it without a full-time nanny and William's support, and even so it can be overwhelming." Elaine is an outgoing, curvaceous woman with soulful eyes whose coolly confident air and quick wit attract attention wherever she goes. She grew up in a "normally neurotic" traditional nuclear family, met William while still in college, and reports that it was love at first sight for both of them. "It was originally William's idea to open up our marriage about five years ago. He's both practical and idealistic and believes that if we want to continue creating a great relationship for the rest of our lives, we need to allow each other freedom. I agreed to give it a try." Elaine and William started by exploring swinging, but before long, she fell in love with Timothy. Elaine says that they made some good friends in the swing community but that she and William soon tired of recreational sex and realized that they preferred relationships with more substance. "We realized polyamory is a better fit for us than swinging. William has fallen for a few single women, but they've all been reluctant to dive in with a married man. I'm lucky Timothy is already married and open and happy with things the way they are," she sighs.

Alice is a world apart from Elaine in terms of both geography and life-style. This twenty-seven-year-old single Danish woman lives in Zurich, Switzerland, where she works for a high-tech company. Like Elaine, she's an articulate and creative young woman who knows what she wants from life—and what she doesn't. And one thing she doesn't want is a traditional marriage, not even a polyamorous one. Like many young women, Alice began having monogamous relationships but after several painful breakups reached the conclusion that perhaps the problem was less with her ability to relate and more with the form the relationships were supposed to take and resolved to abstain from monogamy. "It was never about the sex for me or even gender," Alice says. "Sex wasn't the problem; it was more the weird relationship dynamics." She now has a small circle of friends and lovers and is much happier. She says she wants to have children some day but within a tribal context rather than with a specific partner.

Paula is a youthful and energetic woman in her mid-fifties who was born in New York. She's been married to Max for twenty years and lived with him for four years before their marriage. Both had had some experience with open relationships before meeting. Max had previously been in an open marriage for eight years, and Paula had dated a man who also had another girlfriend. Paula recalls that "we didn't really have a position on it," and monogamy wasn't something they discussed before moving in together. Nevertheless, they soon found themselves meeting people and being invited to sexually open parties. Paula says that at first she was the one who was interested in having other partners, but Max was willing to go along. "The men would always be all over me. I was cute and hot, and I got a lot of attention. Max was a little shy and retiring, and he'd get jealous. I'd tell him he should be happy for me. I was having a good time, but looking back I can see that I unintentionally caused him a lot of pain, I just wasn't sensitive to his feelings. After a while I got involved in a long-term relationship with another man and toned it down at the parties, and that made it easier on Max. At the same time, we started taking classes on sex and relationship and learned some good communication skills as well as sexual techniques. Max and I decided to get married at this point, and my lover was also married, so the four of us hung out a lot for a few years, although Max and the other woman didn't really connect all that well, and eventually we stopped seeing each other. But the whole experience helped us realize that we were polyamorous. We liked how it felt and felt it was working for us."

Paula has had the freedom to explore other relationships in part because she chose not to have any children, and she's always worked on her own creative projects. Her next boyfriend moved in with them, and for the next four years, Max enjoyed a series of short-term relationships with many different women while Paula focused on the two main guys in her life. After she broke up with her boyfriend, both Paula and Max were "single" for a year and used to joke that even though it was just the two of them, they still felt they were poly. Before long, Paula and Max were living in a foursome with her lover Henry and Max's lover Margaret. Although Henry and Margaret didn't get along well and Max was still troubled by jealousy, Paula still felt it was a positive experience overall. Margaret left after a year, and the others stayed together as a threesome for several more years, but eventually Max decided it was time for Henry to find a woman of his own. Henry chose a woman who thought she wanted polyamory but who later decided she couldn't handle it, so Henry and his new wife moved into their own home. Not long after this, Paula met David, and they've been together for the past ten years. David also has another girlfriend who is married. Meanwhile, Max has had relationships with several other women and rarely experiences jealousy anymore. Paula says that she and Max have stayed together all these years because they enjoy each other's company, they're sexually compatible and considerate, respectful, and appreciative of each other. "He takes really good care of me," Paula reports, "and we believe in investing in our relationship. No one person can fulfill all your needs. There are things he wants that I can't give him, but I can set him free to find those things elsewhere."

Paula acknowledges that she had a very traumatic childhood and feels it's been profoundly healing for her to have had so many good experiences with men. "I'm a complex person," she says, "and it's hard to find everything I want in just one man." Part of what Paula is looking for with other men is someone who enjoys sharing her bondage, discipline, dominance, submission, and sadomasochism fantasy play, which doesn't appeal to Max at all. She also values the opportunity to have interacted so closely with Max's lovers but admits that a lot of the women have had problems with her. "They'd fall in love with Max, and they'd get mad at me for no apparent reason. They'd get irrational. Maybe there's something I'm not seeing, but I don't think it has anything to do with me. I've had to learn not to take it personally and to respect them where they're at and give them space if that's what they want."

Paula suspects that she's underestimated how hard it is for people to accept polyamory. "I just want everyone to be one big happy family, but it seems someone is always throwing daggers at me. Why can't we all be friends?" But the hardest part of polyamory for Paula is the need to constantly be juggling a complicated schedule of who is spending time with whom. "It's one never-ending decision making process. Sometimes I just don't know who I want to be with, or I want it all, I want to be with my husband and my boyfriend. It's hard to make plans with others because I don't know where I'll be, with who, or when. If Max was not out of town so often for his job, I don't know how I would manage at all."

Rainah defied her conservative father by leaving her native Austria and going to live in the community that gathered around Bhagwan Shree Rajneesh in Pune, India, while she was still a teenager. She later followed Bhagwan (now known as Osho) to the new ashram in Oregon. After the new ashram dissolved, she moved to the San Francisco Bay Area along with many other sanyasins and enrolled in a nursing program at the local community college. Now in her mid-forties, she's an attractive, vivacious woman who has never married or had children, though she's had several long-term relationships. She runs her own successful practice as a nurse practitioner and appears organized, competent, and down to earth.

Rainah is grateful to have been in the presence of this unconventional guru in the early days before the publicity about sexual experimentation at the ashram and his collection of Rolls Royce limos made headlines worldwide. "He was a genius with words and with energy," she reminisces. "He touched something in all of us with the love that he exuded and the razor-sharp way he could see right through you. I remember my first darshan (private audience) with him. I was a teenager and quite self-centered and full of myself. Just the way he looked at me I got that there was no one there to be impressed. It was a huge puncture to my personality. He blew me away instantly." In those days, in the late 1970s, it was still under 100 people, about three-quarters wealthy professional westerners in their thirties and forties, about one-quarter young Indians, Rainah reports. "It didn't matter what people did or what the community did later on, it never affected my view of Osho. It was just a giant lesson to never give our power away. Power corrupts, and absolute power corrupts absolutely, as the old saying goes."

Osho was working largely with breaking down the egos of the westerners; and there were many naked encounter groups with permission to break all taboos. Osho supported "taking the lid off sexually" and encouraged sexual experimentation because he wanted his followers to move through the cultural obsession with sexuality so that they could go on to love and meditation. "In his presence, everything would come up—any self hatred, anything you were holding on to, anything you didn't accept about yourself. . . . Sex was such a small part of what was going on. So much was being broken down. Sure there was jealousy, but it was a small thing relative to everything else." After some time, people started to become more "natural." Rainah recalls that by sixteen she had had many sexual experiences but eventually settled down for a time with an Indian boyfriend. "It wasn't a decision," she says, "it just happened that way."

For Rainah, the sexual experiences, even for a hormone-driven teenager, were much less significant than the energy darshans with Osho. The women would meet on the marble terrace in the garden outside his house in the evening, and he would "touch certain places where something needed to move. It was not a physical touch, the only physical contact would be sometimes a finger on the third eye (between the eyebrows). Osho would be surrounded by a few women who were able to amplify his energy, and he would energetically work with several other women in one evening. Some women would swoon or gyrate or make sounds, and it was all very sensual. To an observer, it would have looked like a strange kind of orgy."

"I could die any time now and not feel like I missed anything" is how Rainah describes her experience of darshan with Osho. "Osho said that some people are on a path of relationship and others on a path of meditation, but I feel that for me it's both. In some of his talks, Osho said you could only go very deeply if you stayed with one person, but you have to remember that he was always talking to a specific person who may have asked him a question. And he could say something one day and say just the opposite the next day."

Until recently, Rainah was in a ten-year relationship with Devesh, who was an Osho sanyasin. Devesh divided his time between Rainah and another woman who he'd been living with for twenty years, and he also had a number of other partners during this time, while Rainah chose to have no other sexual partners. She says she went deeper into the practice of sex as meditation and healing with Devesh than she ever had before and at this point does not go into a sexual relationship without first taking the time to see how it may impact her and whether it will be in the best interest for both her and her potential lover—unless, of course, it's one of those "really clear and clean" situations with no potential for drama that is just pure fun, she adds.

Over the years, Rainah has come to realize that she'll never be able to say ahead of time whether she will be monogamous with a given person and even then that it could change over time depending on what's happening in her life. "I'm neither for monogamy nor against it," she says. "I still have a romantic streak, and I used to always be asking myself, am I polyamorous, or am I monogamous? Now I'm comfortable with knowing that I'm neither; it's just very moment to moment. It's no longer a mental decision. It will change depending on who I'm with. I can see the good in both monogamy and polyamory. I just have to keep being real with myself, owning my conditioning and not mistaking that for who I really am."

All these women are very different from each other and represent very different ways of expressing femininity as well as practicing polyamory. Nevertheless, they're all strong, creative, independent women who are determined to make their own choices in life whether or not they've married. Some find in polyamory an effective way to address personal issues that might make monogamy difficult or impossible; others are simply attracted to a more expanded and authentic means of self-expression.

QUINTESSENTIAL POLYAMOROUS MEN

Polyamorous men are just as diverse a group as polyamorous women, but one thing they seem to have in common is that however traditionally masculine they may or may not be and whatever their age, if they are hetero- or bisexual, they place a strong value on women's sexual autonomy and have a deep respect for the feminine. Usually, they were raised by mothers who were strongly independent, even in cultures or life circumstances where this was not common. These are men who embody a sensual appreciation for life, and while they may be critical of patriarchy, they are strikingly proactive in effectively creating satisfying lives for themselves in a strongly masculine way.

Ned is now sixty-nine years old and retired two years ago from a successful business career. Prior to this, he served as a military pilot in Vietnam, which he looks back on as a grand adventure and the best time in his life even though he was philosophically opposed to the war. As he saw it, he was stuck in a bad situation but figured he might as well make the most of it. Ned is a self-described intensity junkie who enjoyed the fast-paced excitement of evading enemy aircraft and exploring the bars and women of Bangkok as much as he later enjoyed juggling several multi-million-dollar deals at a time. He was concerned that he'd be bored and restless after retirement despite many activities, including a season pass for his favorite football team, biking, hatha yoga, meditation, surfing, and adventure travel. He needn't have worried. Relationships have become his new avocation.

At the time of his retirement, Ned was no stranger to nonmonogamy. He'd explored swinging in the 1970s with his second wife. He enjoyed the socializing and the sex, but after their divorce, he looked around at the people he knew and noticed that none of the ones who'd had open marriages were still together. He decided to give monogamy a try and was happily married to Marjorie for thirteen years. "I'm pretty sure Marjorie would never have considered anything nonmonogamous, but it never came up. I was happy with her, there was no need to discuss it." Ned says they'd still be together today had she not died after a sudden heart attack. He was devastated by his wife's death but after a year of mourning decided it was time to start dating again.

After several short-lived relationships Ned bumped into Faith at a party, and they've been inseparable ever since. Ned and Faith first met at a swing party back in the 1970s and became friends and lovers. Their children were best friends, and Ned had been buddies with Faith's ex-husband, but they lost touch when Faith remarried and moved to another state. For the first several years, Ned and Faith were busy with their work and their new romance. They shared an occasional sexual adventure with another old lover, but Ned remembered the soap operas of open relationships twenty years earlier and felt cautious about going there again. Gradually, he discovered that in his absence polyamory had come into its own and that swinging had dramatically changed. "People seem more mature and more realistic and just generally better prepared for a nonmonogamous lifestyle than they used to be," he observed. Before his retirement, Ned and Faith limited their involvement with others mostly to a few old friends, but now, with more leisure time, they have regular dates with two couples in their late fifties who they met at swing parties. Ned says that with one couple it's purely sex; with the other there's the possibility of a deeper relationship. "They're both very intelligent and interesting, but they're newbies, so we're taking it very slow."

Ned also has intimate friendships with three other women. Jacqueline is in her early fifties and coping with a sexless marriage and has a "don't ask, don't tell" agreement with her husband. She has a regular bimonthly date with Ned and Faith (who is bisexual and thoroughly enjoys the threesomes Ned arranges). Ama, who is a refuge from the war-torn Middle East, and Satya, an Indian woman who was raised in London, are both single mothers in their thirties who enjoy the sense of expanded family as well as the erotic connection with Ned and Faith. Ned's grandchildren live thousands of miles away, and he likes including children into his life. While he's clear that he's just doing what he enjoys and is good at, Ned also gets satisfaction from knowing that he's providing sexual gratification and emotional support for women who might otherwise have to do without.

How does a man pushing seventy manage five part-time women and one primary partner? Ned says it just happens by itself. "I didn't think getting older was going to be like this," he confesses. "It's just incredible. I feel like a sultan. If I'd known it would be like this, I would have retired sooner. And life just keeps getting better." Ned is a high-energy, athletic man with a can-do attitude and a rare appreciation for both the safe, practical, predictable material side of life and the edgy, dangerous aliveness of new people, new places, and new experiences.

Ned's parents divorced in the 1950s when he was in elementary school. He spent most weekends with his father, but his mother, who was a feisty schoolteacher, openly had a series of lovers in the era before women's liberation. Ned is emotionally intelligent and a good communicator, and while he's comfortable in the world of men, he says that most of his friends are women because it's been hard to establish close friendships with other men. His strong alpha persona may present a challenge to relating intimately with other men while making him a magnet for women, and that's just fine with his fiery bisexual partner.

Graham is half Ned's age and has a more androgenous appearance but also enjoys the affection of several women. He was born in a working-class neighborhood in London thirty-five years ago but now divides his time between several European cities where he is developing both his art career and his intimate relationships. He says that he began having spontaneous spiritual experiences as a young boy and as he grew older began seeking ways to understand the other dimensions that had been revealed to him. His quest led him to India, where he studied yoga and meditation, and he began to be interested in ways he could build a life based on spirituality. Graham remembers first exploring the idea of non-monogamy as a teenager. "I was seeing a girl in a casual way when I met another girl who I also liked. As the original relationship was casual, I felt that it wouldn't be an issue to also explore the possibility of being with the new girl. However, I always had a belief in being open and honest, so I explained to the new girl the situation with the first. She was okay with it at first but then felt it wasn't for her. I continued to see the first girl, and we moved on to explore the possibilities of nonmonogamy together, including a triad situation a little while after. In fact, we continued to see each other for nearly a decade, and I am still friends with both of them some eighteen years later."

While still in his early twenties, Graham began to see a young woman who would turn out to be a primary partner for ten years. At first, they decided they would have an open relationship, but before long, the lack of trust and communication led them to shift to monogamy. Graham commented that "the fact that we had to do this, in a sense to hold on to the relationship, was a sign of the future problems that led to our split. When we did finally split and she met a new guy, I felt a sense of *compersion* for the first time. I was genuinely happy for her and felt that I too could get back to a sense of who I really was away from the limitations I had built around myself and her." Shortly afterward, he met his first openly polyamorous partner.

Graham continues, "We started off as a couple, but later I began to see her ex-partner. About eight months after that, we developed into a triad-type relationship. However, I don't put any limits on how I or my partners should love—other than being safe, honest and open. Also around the same time, I became involved with a young woman with a small child. She was still involved with the father, and we explored the idea of her maintaining her relationship with him as the father and me as her lover, but unfortunately he was not able to accept the situation despite us spending time together and enjoying each other's company."

Graham has recently begun two new relationships but says it's too early to tell how they will develop. One is with a fellow artist who identifies as polyamorous, and the other is new to all this and isn't sure what she wants. Graham feels that "my intimate relationships and connections with people form in a very organic way. I tend to focus on long-term bonds, and most of my lovers remain my close friends, although the exact configuration of my intimate partners may change."

Graham says that although he was drawn to multiple partners from an early age, more recently he's come to appreciate that polyamory is an extension of the theme of unity consciousness, which has also led him to actively involve himself with spiritual, political, and social issues. Polyamory got more interesting to Graham when he "started to see that freeing up the way you love and holding your heart open to the possibilities that life may bring is a very powerful way to live. Being able to look at a partner and feel an outpouring of emotion and love for them, but without a need to be possessive or controlling, is genuinely life changing. My interest in equality, LGBTQ, and feminist ideas also seemed to be given greater power by exploring polyamory or relationship anarchy. When I first identified as polyamorous, I had already recently become vegan as an extension of my values, so becoming open to greater loving possibilities seemed the logical next step towards greater compassion, awareness, and understanding."

Daniel, like Graham, is part of a new generation who are taking on leadership positions in the world of polyamory. Daniel is a twenty-three-year-old Portuguese graduate student in communication who lives in Lisbon with his divorced mother and his beautiful girlfriend, Sofia. For the past year, Daniel and Sofia have been in a triad with another young woman, and Daniel is also exploring a new relationship. Daniel was raised in the Portugal countryside in a very conservative family of Jehovah's Witnesses. He describes himself as a "miniature adult" with few friends his own age. His parents divorced while he was in grade school, and he moved to a rough urban neighborhood with his mother. He seems relieved to have escaped the religious atmosphere, but as a short, chubby bookworm, he was frequently bullied. Partly as a result of his direct experience of the dark side of masculinity and being surrounded by women while growing up, he's gravitated both toward feminist theory and toward women for his social needs. He has very few male friends.

"It bothers me that I have been granted such power and benefits just for being male. I dislike the fact that my sex is equivalent to a whole history of submission and aggression," he explains. "Male friendship usually has an aggressive edge, with which I'm not comfortable and a lack of any psychological and emotional intimacy—not to mention any nonaggressive physical contact—which definitely doesn't suit me. So I tend to form more meaningful bonds with people of the opposite sex."

Daniel says that his childhood experiences of discrimination, along with a strong sense of fairness and social justice, have led him to take a stand for what he believes in. He's appeared on Portuguese television and given interviews to the press as well as being active in the local polyamorous community. "Discrimination is based on false perceptions, and the deconstruction of any form of discrimination is the deconstruction of all forms of discrimination. And one of the most insidious forms of discrimination and imbalance is gender based," Daniel informed me. "I don't think I'd be happy in a relationship with someone that wasn't my equal. It would seem oppressive to me, and it would teach me nothing."

As usual, I'm awed by the way this generation is able to go straight to the heart of the matter, but Daniel is less sanguine. "As for my generation, I wish I could be so optimistic. Yes, things are changing. Yes, gender imbalances are starting to fade. But not as quickly or as deeply as I'd like. And there are lots of contradictory behaviors. Sexual experimentation goes hand in hand with polyphobia and mononormative and possessive relationships. Romantic love seems like the Holy Grail of serial monogamy, elevated to the notion of a state of pure nirvana but always out of reach, always elusive. There's a frenzied hunt for the perfect relationship. I fear a society where an educated twenty-year-old woman can say, without the hint of a doubt, that it is impossible to love more than one person at the same time while she herself has behaviors that society would deem promiscuous and sinful. Then again, I've seen lots of people gladly accepting such things quite nicely. So, no, I don't actually think my generation will make such a difference, not in the short run at least. We need to be disillusioned first, beyond hope, before we are willing to think outside the box."

PERSONALITY TRAITS AND POLYAMORY

Polyamory can be a complex and demanding lovestyle. I often tell people that it requires a higher level of self-awareness and interpersonal skills than monogamy. Research on the personality traits shared by most polyamorous people has yet to be conducted, but many observers have noticed that certain characteristics are common among those choosing polyamory. Many of these traits are apparent in all the personalities profiled in this chapter.

A Talent for Intimate Relating

Perhaps the most basic trait found among those attracted to and successful in polyamorous relationships is that they have a talent for intimate relationships. Some people have a gift for music, and others are natural athletes. If you have a gift for connecting with others, for giving and receiving affection, and if you're empathic and compassionate and enjoy sharing life's pleasures and sorrows with a group of people, then you have a talent for relating intimately. Without this talent, it can be a struggle to handle even one meaningful relationship. People who have a gift for relating find that they have the capacity for opening their hearts to many and greatly enjoy becoming involved in other people's lives. This talent sometimes leads people into one of the helping professions—nursing, psychotherapy, teaching, or social work. Such people make good managers, community organizers, parents, and sometimes politicians.

High Self-Esteem

Any intimate relationship is difficult without a sense of self-worth, which is not dependent on validation from someone else. Relying on a partner to make you feel desirable, special, or lovable inevitably leads to wanting to control and possess this source of positive regard. A partner's attraction to someone else, whether or not it's acted on, will be perceived as a threat if you need constant reassurance that you're okay. It takes plenty of self-confidence to be willing to share your lovers with others, secure in the knowledge that you won't be found lacking in some essential quality. High self-esteem makes it possible to face the unknown without excessive fears. It transforms problems into challenges that can be met with courage, persistence, and creativity. Even though the security, predictability, and control that monogamy seems to offer often turns out to be an illusion, polyamory tends to put people in the fire of uncertainty on a regular basis. People who've developed a confident awareness that they're capable of riding out whatever life brings their way are more open to surrendering to the flow of love.

Ability to Multitask

Some people function best doing one thing at a time with no distractions. Others find it easy to track several different processes at once by shifting back and forth as needed. Such people often prefer the variety and stimulation of having a broader focus. People who can juggle tasks, projects, and quickly changing priorities usually have the ability to juggle several intimate relationships as well without dropping the ball.

A Love for Intensity

Polyamory often means more activity, more interaction, more energy, more interests, more change, more obligations, more communication, more coordination, more time, more everything. Long-term monogamous couples may find that in between developmental crises and periods of rapid growth, there are long uneventful stretches, but with more people involved something is bound to be happening with someone most of the time. People who practice a style of polyamory that involves more than two people spending time together, whether in or out of bed, find that the combined presence of an intimate, no-barriers group of people creates a definite intensity of its own.

Appreciation for Diversity

Every group or family needs to come to terms with differences among its members. People who need everyone in their intimate circle to be exactly like them in order to feel comfortable are going to experience greater and greater levels of frustration in this endeavor the more partners they have. While relationships work best when partners share common values, part of the joy of polyamory is recognizing and supporting each person's unique qualities.

Communication Skills

Communication skills can make or break any intimate relationship, and they are not limited to the ability to use words well (although that helps). Awareness of nonverbal cues and body language is just as important in navigating the complexities of out-of-the-box relationships as the ability to express desires, needs, resentments, appreciation, and hurt feelings and to effectively negotiate win–win solutions to conflicts.

An Independent Streak

People who have good boundaries and value their autonomy are often unwilling to allow a partner to take over control of their hearts or their genitals. They usually prefer relationships that acknowledge their right to feel attraction to others, although they may be willing to negotiate on how these attractions will be dealt with if they also have a team spirit.

Team Spirit

While most people attracted to polyamory value their autonomy, independence alone makes it difficult to cooperate with others over time.
When independence is combined with a team spirit, it sets the stage for
a win–win style, which can create a powerful synergy with others. Polyamorous people tend to recognize that working for the good of the whole
group will benefit them more in the long run than an exclusive focus on
their own personal agendas.

Commitment to Growth

Polyamory is an inherently demanding lovestyle, and as long as most
people continue to be socialized for monogamy, it will continue to be even
more challenging. Relating intimately to more than one person at a time
provides more mirroring and less opportunity to blame "the other" for your
own dysfunctional programming. For people who want to use their relationships as opportunities for learning and healing, polyamory presents a
valuable way of accelerating growth. Although some people see polyamory
as an escape from intimacy, in a committed polyamorous relationship it's
much harder to "hide."

Sex Positive

While some people are attracted to polyamory because they have a high
sex drive, they're looking for a solution to a mismatch in desire levels or
sexual orientation, or they're simply hoping to "spice up" an existing long-
term relationship, polyamory is about more than "just" sex. On the other
hand, people who are uncomfortable with their own or other people's
sexuality usually don't want the kind of exposure to additional partners that
polyamory inevitably brings with it, even if the actual sexual encounters are
always one-on-one and take place at a safe distance.

Flexible, Creative, Spontaneous

Polyamory makes it much more difficult to maintain an illusion of predictability and control. As anyone who has children knows, chaos better
describes the complexities of multiple, interacting individuals. Those who
enjoy the spontaneity of not knowing exactly what's going to happen next

and who like finding creative solutions to unanticipated developments are more likely to choose polyamory than those who have a strong need for control. Flexibility makes it possible for a group to share power through situational leadership and maximize the potential for synergy, which is much less in a dyad than a larger group.

High Intelligence

I certainly wouldn't characterize all polyamorous people as geniuses or monogamous people as being unintelligent, but numerous observers have commented that polyamorous people tend to be far above the norms on many dimensions of intelligence, including but not limited to emotional intelligence. Perhaps those who are more inclined to think for themselves and are better able to assess each situation on its own merits are more likely to end up polyamorous, or perhaps one needs the extra capacity to handle all the complexities polyamory can present. Whatever the explanation, there's a strong correlation.

Accountability

Every relationship works better when people can be counted on to do what they say they're going to do and take responsibility for cleaning up any messes that result from occasional lapses. In polyamorous relationships, one person's lack of responsibility impacts many others. It is the lack of self-responsibility and accountability among many of the free-spirited but immature and unprepared early adopters of polyamory that led to its reputation as an "unworkable" lifestyle. As more mainstream people who have learned the importance of accountability and self-awareness in the business arena or in rigorous spiritual training discover polyamory, I predict that they will have greater success than has been seen in the past.

THE ALPHA PROBLEM

Every relationship journey involves finding a way to resolve what is commonly known as the power struggle. When I work with couples or other groups, one of the first questions I ask is, "Who's the boss in this relationship?" Of all the thousands of clients who have sought my help in getting through their relationship challenges, there has never been one who didn't know who had the last word, although some are hesitant to be so direct. It's extremely rare for partners to have different perceptions in this area as well. They may report that it's changed over time, that each is in charge of different domains, or that this is a constant source of conflict, but they always know the score. In old-paradigm relationships, complementary pairings of one dominant and one submissive individual or, in the case of polyandry or polygyny, a spouse who is submissive to the patriarch or matriarch but dominant over the cowives or cohusbands is the rule.

Sexual intimacy thrives on polarity, and when the sexual interaction goes deep enough, it involves a reversal of this polarity. That is, the active becomes receptive, and the receptive becomes active, harmonizing the divergent energies each partner brings. This takes place regardless of the genders of the partners or their sexual orientation. In a triad or larger grouping where two same-gender partners are primarily heterosexual, the energetic exchange is rarely full enough to reconcile the power struggle. One strong alpha leader, whether male or female, can sometimes exert enough control to keep all the others in line, but two alphas in one family often spells pandemonium, and, in fact, this configuration rarely even occurs. On the other hand, two or more submissive types can sometimes "gang up" on an alpha and tilt the power balance, sometimes driving the alpha out of the group only to find that the group falls apart without the strong leadership of the alpha.

Two or more alphas can harmoniously coexist only when one or both are essentially beyond being ruled by unconscious or semiconscious egoic drives. In fact, all relationships work much better when the personalities or egos take a back seat to something higher. For humanist agnostics or atheists, this "something higher" can be the good of the whole or a set of values or a respected leader. For those spiritually or religiously inclined, it can be the Divine, truth, the higher self, Atman, existence, the guru in human form, or whatever metaphor is preferred. In a couple whose dominant and submissive poles are complementary or in a group with one dominant personality and several submissive types, transcending the ego is not critical for stable and harmonious relationships. In the new paradigm of polyamory, where the intention is to bring forth and honor the inner wisdom of each person, chaos and conflict will reign if what is brought forth are egoic demands for control masquerading as truth and love.

6

THE CHALLENGE OF JEALOUSY

Jealousy is not unique to polyamory, nor is it the only emotional challenge encountered in polyamorous relating, but it is certainly the number one difficulty for most people who venture beyond monogamy. The mere thought of jealousy is enough to motivate some people to exchange vows of lifelong sexual fidelity, while others do exactly the opposite and seek jealousy insurance by making sure that they always have a spare lover in the wings. In the end, the only way out of jealousy is through it, and polyamory certainly offers abundant opportunities to make this journey. As popular author Thomas Moore put it, "We may have to let jealousy have its way with us and do its job of reorienting fundamental values. Its pain comes, at least in part, from opening up to unexplored territory and letting go of old familiar truths in the face of unknown and threatening possibilities."[1] Moore was not specifically referring to polyamory or even sexual jealousy, which is known to be particularly intense and powerful, but his remarks are right on target.

While the somatic experience of jealousy is remarkably consistent no matter what the context, there is one obvious difference between jealousy in monogamous relationships and jealousy in polyamorous ones. In a monogamous relationship, where choice of a mate is clearly an either/or proposition, jealousy may be a reasonable strategy to keep others away from your partner or to discourage your partner from pursuing others. If your partner falls for someone else, it's a realistic threat to your continued marital bliss. In polyamory, other lovers are not necessarily a danger, although, as we shall see, they can be. When partners agree that including others would enhance their lives, unyielding jealousy and possessiveness can become obstacles to their ongoing happiness rather than functioning to protect a dyadic bond.

Despite its pervasiveness in human experience as reflected in literature and film, jealousy has been one of the least studied of all human emotions. It doesn't even appear in the index of Daniel Goleman's groundbreaking book on emotional literacy *Emotional Intelligence*.[2] Let's begin by exploring the nature of jealousy before moving on to consider where it comes from, what messages it brings us, and how it can best be managed.

WHAT IS JEALOUSY, AND WHY DO WE DREAD IT?

Jealousy has gotten surprisingly little attention from researchers, and most of the research that's been done addresses the attitudes, thoughts, and behaviors associated with jealousy rather than with the neurophysiological correlates or the experiential nature of the emotion itself. Neuroimaging is only in the early stages of its investigation of jealousy. In a 2006 study reported in *NeuroImage*, Japanese neuroscientist Hidehiko Takahashi found some significant sex differences in the neural response to statements depicting sexual and emotional infidelity. In men, jealousy activates the amygdala and hypothalamus, regions rich in testosterone receptors and involved in sexual and aggressive behavior. In women, thoughts of emotional infidelity activate the posterior superior temporal sulcus, a region implicated in the detection of intention, deception, and trustworthiness as well as violation of social norms. Takahashi interpreted the greater activation elicited by emotional infidelity in females as evidence that they're particularly sensitive to changes in a partner's mind. Perhaps his findings account for the greater tendency of men to react to the sexual act itself rather than its emotional implications.

Most researchers agree that on a cognitive-behavioral level, sexual jealousy is a reaction to a partner's real or imagined experience with a third party and that jealousy is most likely to occur in a person who is both dependent and insecure.[3] My own clinical observation based on working with thousands of people struggling with jealousy is that jealousy most often arises when a person's need for control is threatened. This may or may not coincide with dependency and low self-esteem.

What I find most fascinating about jealousy is the actual bodily sensations and internal thoughts and energetic events that create the experience of jealousy. People commonly describe jealous sensations as gut wrenching, churning, agitating, arousing, and overpoweringly unpleasant. While different people become jealous for different reasons and in differing circumstances, the actual physical feelings are remarkably consistent from person to person, although they may vary in intensity. Even a low level of jealousy is usually uncomfortable enough that most people will try to distract themselves or take some action to eliminate the perceived cause of their jealousy. Consequently, it is only in body-centered psychotherapy with a nonjudgmental therapist or in some kinds of spiritual practices, such as vipassana meditation or self-inquiry, that people are likely to explore the experience of jealousy without immediately trying to escape it. Early on, I realized that in order to really understand what jealousy is and how it operates and to what end, I would have to examine my own inner process. If you too want to understand jealousy, I invite you to do the same. The next time the opportunity arises, instead of pushing it away, welcome the chance to investigate the nature of jealousy. Fortunately, I was already quite experienced in being with uncomfortable feelings, and my own jealousy tended toward relatively low intensity, so I was well suited for this endeavor. Here's what I found to be true for myself.

I'm most vulnerable to jealousy when I'm feeling both love and sexual arousal. Love is felt primarily in my heart center, in the center of the chest, as a sensation of expansion or sometimes cracking open or radiating outward. These physical sensations are accompanied by a sense of connection or oneness with others. Sexual arousal arises from the pelvic region as a high-voltage current, heat and tingling from my pelvic floor up into my genitals and lower abdomen, radiating both downward to my toes and upward to the top of my head. Both sensations are very pleasurable and can easily induce a desire to join with another to further increase and disperse the energy. They raise my sensitivity to stimuli of all kinds and at the same time raise my pain threshold. The experience is one of being supercharged or energized and at the same time feeling everything inside me and around me more deeply.

If something then occurs that I think might separate me from my beloved or love object, fear and anger arise within me. The fear is felt as a contraction, a tightening, and a shutting down. The anger is energizing, like sexual arousal, and like sexual arousal, it seeks a release and connection with something outside me, but it also hardens my heart center, contracting it and walling it off. These impulses of contraction and shutting down collide with the already established wave of expansion and opening up. Mind and body are confused. They cannot gracefully contain such duality. Unable to wrap my consciousness around this resounding contradiction, I long to jump out of my skin and call this powerful, churning, open-and-closed-at-the-same-time sensation jealousy. If I stay with it, I find I have a choice. I can channel this energy into further opening my heart, amplifying my arousal, leaving my body, or exploding in anger.

Another way of saying this would be that jealousy can feel like a powerful blend of all emotions at once. Love, sexual arousal, fear, and anger may all be blended together into one gigantic ball of energy that threatens to overwhelm the rational mind. If a single strong emotion has the potential to "hijack" us, as Daniel Goleman puts it in *Emotional Intelligence*, what chance do we stand against jealousy? The key, as in dealing with all emotions, is to notice the early signals of its approach and take appropriate action while we still have our wits about us. But what is an appropriate response to jealousy?

IS JEALOUSY HEALTHY AND INEVITABLE?

Evolutionary psychologist David Buss argues that sexual jealousy is healthy, necessary, and useful. Buss claims that jealousy not only helped ensure that our male ancestors were the biological fathers of their women's offspring and that our female ancestors could rely on the ongoing support of their men but also that it continues to serve the purpose of maintaining sexual exclusivity, igniting sexual passion, and becoming aware of a partner's infidelity.[4]

Traditionally, a psychological distinction has been made between jealousy arising from a known infidelity and an imagined one. The first is considered normal, the second pathological or neurotic. While there are certainly people whose jealous suspicions have absolutely no basis in reality, Buss cites many examples of cases in which a spouse's apparently unfounded jealousy later turns out to have been an accurate intuition of a past, ongoing, or even future affair. But the ability to know when a sexual partner has had an intimate encounter with someone else does not always result in jealousy. Instead, Moore's insight about jealousy being a reaction to unknown and threatening possibilities is more consistent with my own observations as illustrated by the following case history.

Linda and Mark came to me seeking help repairing their sexless marriage. Mark is an attractive, athletic man in his mid-thirties, and Linda is a pretty, somewhat overweight woman a few years older than Mark. Both grew up in the San Francisco Bay Area and began dating each other while in college. When Mark took a semester abroad, they'd decided to open their relationship, and each had other partners without creating any drama between them. Linda had done her best to fulfill Mark's sexual needs for the first eight years they'd been together. While she'd been easily orgasmic, she'd always felt something was lacking in their sexual connection, but she didn't know what it was or how to talk about it. After the birth of their son four years earlier, she'd become increasingly sexually withdrawn and resentful about Mark's sexual demands. Both Linda and Mark were afraid that if they continued as they were, they would end up divorced, an outcome that neither wanted because of their shared commitment to parenting and to a successful business they had started together.

In the course of working with them, I asked each to meet with me separately. When Linda came in alone, she immediately confessed that she was having a secret affair with one of their employees. "I know I should stop seeing Ricky," she moaned, "but I just can't make myself. Sex with Ricky is giving me something I always wanted and could never find with Mark. It's not just sex, it's deep and loving, almost a religious experience. I didn't know it could be like this. I've encouraged Mark to find another woman for sex, but he says he just wants me. The trouble is that I just can't settle for the mechanical sex we were having now that I know there's something else. Thank God he's not the jealous type, or I'd have no choice but to divorce him! The problem is that Ricky is an employee, and that really complicates things."

Meanwhile, Mark began his session by saying, "I think Linda's having an affair. I've hinted around about it, and she plays innocent, but I don't believe her. It really hurts me that she's not telling me about it. I'd be willing to have an open relationship if that's what she wants. I'm scared it would wreck our marriage, but it would be better than cheating." As Mark shared more about his feelings, it became apparent that he really was not jealous. He wanted Linda's love and acceptance, but sharing was not a problem for him. He wasn't really interested in taking on another lover himself because he didn't want the emotional complications, but he didn't want a life without sex either. Mark's parents had had a consensually open marriage, and he'd grown up at ground zero in the heyday of the sexual revolution. Polyamory was not an alien concept for him, but it was not really appealing either. His father was quite a lady's man, and his mother eventually grew tired of her husband's constant womanizing and divorced him. Mark and Linda definitely had marital problems, but jealousy was not one of them.

Buss maintains that sexual jealousy has been a successful means of passing on genetic information, and because of this, today's men and women are prone to jealousy and possessiveness. "Nonjealous men and women are not our ancestors, having been left in the evolutionary dust by rivals with different passionate sensibilities. We all come from a long lineage of ancestors who possessed the dangerous passion,"[5] he asserts. But what about the clever unfaithful who didn't get caught and who may have conceived with nonjealous partners before returning to socially monogamous mates as is so common in the animal kingdom? What about all the DNA lost in murders committed in acts of jealous rage?

Most significantly, what about all the ancestors who either didn't know or didn't care about biological fatherhood? Many experts believe that until the rise of patriarchy about 4,000 years ago, biological fatherhood was not of much interest to humans.[6] This is a very brief time frame in the million or so years of human evolution. In the matrilineal societies that were once dominant, names, titles, and property rights are passed down through the maternal line. To this day, it is the mother, not the father, whose lineage determines whether their baby is Jewish. Well into historical times in many places around the world, the royal line passed from mother to daughter, and even after queens were replaced by kings, the king derived his right to rule from his wife or mother. All these customs point to cultures in which paternity was unimportant socially and emotionally.

Among many indigenous people, children are still regarded as belonging to "the village" rather than either biological parent. In Hawaii, in premissionary times it was customary to accept as kin the children your partner previously or subsequently conceived with another partner. In the old days, jealousy in these situations was rare, but today it is expected. Adoption of children on the basis of affinity, regardless of blood ties, was common and is a tradition even now.[7] Far from being the utopian fantasy that Buss suggests, disregard for paternity, not to mention an absence of lifelong sexual exclusivity, has been the norm throughout most of human evolution, casting doubt on his Darwinian theory of the evolutionary value of jealousy.

Buss admits that jealousy can be dangerous, even fatal. He reports that 13 percent of all homicides occur in domestic violence, and jealousy is almost always involved in domestic violence. The threat of killing or being killed certainly goes a long way toward explaining why jealousy is such a scary prospect. With as many as 50 percent of all married women experiencing spousal violence at some point in their marriages, it's clear that jealousy is pervasive, but it is questionable whether it can be considered healthy. In the research for my doctoral dissertation, I found that the best predictor for whether women in shelters for battered women would leave their abuser or return was whether they believed they had a better alternative than staying in an abusive relationship. In light of this finding, suggesting that jealousy is necessary, useful, and inevitable encourages battered women to tolerate abuse.

In Texas, where Dr. Buss is based, it was permissible until 1974 for a husband to murder his wife and her lover if he discovered them having sex. The law in Texas and in many other places around the world has long considered this kind of "provocation" a defense against prosecution for murder. According to Buss, "Extreme rage upon discovering a wife naked in the arms of another man is something that people everywhere find intuitively comprehensible. Criminal acts that would normally receive harsh prison sentences routinely get reduced when the victim's infidelity is the extenuating circumstance."

As recently as October 2009, a British news article reported that legislators, including former judges, have defeated government plans to stop men from using a wife's infidelity as a partial defense for murdering her. The controversy over the attempted reform has been going on for over a year. The Ministry of Justice said of the Lords vote, "The Government wants to make it clear once and for all, and in statute, that it is unacceptable to kill another person and then claim a partial defense to murder on the grounds of sexual infidelity. . . . The history of the partial-defense of provocation has led to a commonly-held belief that this is a defense which can be abused by men who kill their wives out of sexual jealousy and revenge over infidelity." The equalities minister, Labour's deputy leader, claimed that the proposed change would "end the 'culture of excuses' among men who kill. . . . For centuries the law has allowed men to escape a murder charge in homicide cases by blaming the victim."[8]

"But the move was described as 'astonishing' and 'obnoxious' in the [House of] Lords yesterday as peers rejected an amendment by 99 votes to 84. Crossbencher Lord Neill of Bladen, a retired judge, said, 'We will make ourselves look extraordinarily foolish if we say a jury cannot account of what most people recognise as being the most dominant cause of violence by one individual against another. Every opera you go to, every novel you read has sexual infidelity at some point or other—otherwise they are not worth reading or listening to.'"

"I must confess to being uneasy about a law which so diminishes the significance of sexual infidelity," Lord Phillips of Worth Matravers, the senior law lord, said recently in response to the proposals.[9]

Clearly, there are some in the British parliament who recognize the power of law as well as cultural expectations to shape behavioral norms, but conservatives and liberals are not in agreement about what those norms should be.

Buss admits, "Excessive jealousy can be extraordinarily destructive. But moderate jealousy, not an excess or an absence, signals commitment"—true perhaps in Texas but not necessarily in California. Mark and Linda were as committed to their marriage as any young couple is likely to be these days. Divorce was just not an option they even wanted to think about, although in my opinion it deserved their consideration, but extramarital sex definitely was not a taboo for them. The absence of jealousy in this case was the very thing keeping their marriage together. The question we should be asking is not what can jealousy can do for you or your genetic material but rather what the result is of the belief that jealousy is a good thing, that it's evidence of love or, at least, commitment, as Buss says.

Science has been invoked many times in the past to defend beliefs—and laws—that are now recognized to be not only unsupported by objective evidence but also harmful and dangerous to individuals and to society as a whole. If jealousy is indeed "hardwired," does this mean it's an evolutionary advantage and that it's inevitable? And if it is inevitable, does this mean that monogamy is the best solution, or are there other ways to manage jealousy? We'll address all these questions later on, but for now let's take a look at whether jealousy is genetically or culturally programmed.

NATURE VERSUS NURTURE

As we have seen, people often argue about whether human beings are naturally jealous as a result of our biological heritage or whether jealousy is acquired through cultural conditioning and personal experiences. This issue turns out to more readily fit a "both/and" model than an "either/or" approach. Most likely, people are prone to jealousy because of a combination of acquired beliefs and genetically programmed reactions. The genetic component may well influence whether an individual experiences low-, moderate-, or high-intensity jealousy, but the nagging question remains, how much is nature and how much is nurture?

Since we can't change our nature, a more meaningful question might be, is it possible to overcome jealousy and its destructive effects, or does choosing polyamory imply signing up for a lifetime of jealous agony and melodramatic crises as some people fear? Other important questions to ask are these: How does jealousy affect me, and what can I do about it? Must I feel ashamed of my jealous feelings, or can I accept them as normal and natural without giving them undue importance?

Nearly everyone in our monogamous society learns early in life that spouses have exclusive rights. We are conditioned to believe that if our beloved is interested in someone else, we may be replaced. But this expectation of loss is learned, not hardwired, in both men and women. Imagine a culture in which your partner's attraction to another signified opportunities for greater pleasure, intimacy, and support. Would jealousy occur in this context? As we saw in the previous section, people who are raised in cultures, such as premissionary Hawaii, or subcultures, such as post–Summer of Love San Francisco, where sexual inclusivity is not necessarily a threat and jealousy is not expected, may have different programming than those raised in an environment where an affair is considered an excuse for murder.

My own belief is that while humans have an innate territorial instinct as do other animals, we must learn to view our lovers and spouses as territory or possessions that can be owned like property and that we have a right to control. In other words, jealousy, like other emotions, has definite physiological roots, but the stimuli that trigger jealousy are almost entirely culturally determined. If we look at the behavior of our closest primate relatives, bonobo chimpanzees,[10] we find that both males and females have numerous sex partners, and this doesn't seem to create much conflict within the group. In fact, it appears that bonobos utilize sexual activity to defuse potential conflicts, for example, by sharing sexually prior to dividing up food.

Nevertheless, humans have such a long history of accepting sexual jealousy as inevitable that it's difficult to simply talk ourselves out of it. Cultural programming may not be in our genes, but it operates at an unconscious level that cannot be easily shifted by rational thought. Still, by choosing a belief system that considers jealousy to be an inescapable part of our nature, we resign ourselves to allowing jealousy to control us. If instead we choose to believe that jealousy is learned, we open up the possibility of freeing ourselves from its tyranny.

JEALOUSY IS NOT BETRAYAL

Robert shared the following vivid dream with me. He was helping his friend Denise pack her belongings for an upcoming move. She invited him to make love with her. They were in bed when a large man burst into the room, raging and agitated. Robert was frightened and hid under the sheets, but the man knew he was there. Robert hadn't seen this man before but guessed he might be Denise's husband or boyfriend. Eventually, the man left, and Robert and Denise continued packing. They were moving her boxes into a garage or warehouse on a large concrete slab when the man reappeared and lunged at Robert, trying to strangle him. Robert sat on a box and extended his leg toward the approaching man, flinging him through the air. The man landed on his head, which smashed open on the concrete. Robert and Denise stared at the dead body in horror and disbelief. Robert had only been defending himself and had not intended to kill the man. Denise told him that they would have to find a way to make it look like an accident.

Many people might see this dream as a story about jealousy, but it could just as easily be a dream about betrayal told from the uncommonly heard perspective of "the other man." In fact, much of the violence associated with jealousy could be more accurately attributed to the betrayal with which it's often confused.

The primary issue in jealousy is fear of losing something, whether that's exclusive sexual access, love, attention, reputation, self-esteem, or any of the jealousy triggers we'll talk about later in this chapter. This threat of losing something important to the ego is scary enough for most people without mixing in an overlay of lies, withholds, and half-truths. Feelings of betrayal arise when trust has been shaken because of broken agreements, deception, or a perceived breach of faith. Because so many people are dishonest about their attraction to others or unilaterally break monogamous commitments to have secret affairs, jealousy and betrayal are often linked together.

In the previously described dream, Robert is apparently an innocent bystander, naively helping a friend and not intending to harm anyone. Denise may or may not have anticipated the intrusion of the raging man, and we don't know the history of her relationship with him, but it seems that her taking a lover was not a negotiated agreement. Did she secretly take a lover to avoid a confrontation with her possessive husband? Or did she betray both men by staging the encounters that led to the death of the husband? Was the husband reacting to her moving out, to the sexual interlude, or both? Why does she suggest a cover-up to make it look like an accident when it apparently *was* an accident? The confusion and unanswered questions are typical of a betrayal scenario but need not be part of jealousy that arises in an atmosphere of full disclosure.

I once had a lover who felt both betrayed and jealous of my attraction to another man even though we had a very clear agreement to practice polyamory. He'd agreed to polyamory and thought it was what he wanted, but he still had the unconscious belief that loving more than one person at a time was wrong and evidence of unfaithfulness. If I really loved him, how could I be open to someone else? It was more of a shock to him than to me that the jealous thoughts and feelings he thought he'd transcended were still alive in him. His sense of betrayal turned out to be impossible to resolve, even though the jealousy quickly faded when it became obvious I wasn't going to leave him for this other man.

Conversely, Izzie betrayed his lover Amelia by lying about his illicit affair with Sally and then labeled Amelia's upset as jealousy. When he then urged Amelia to get over her jealousy so that the couple could embark on an open relationship, he greatly impeded both Amelia's healing process and any prospect of transitioning to polyamory. Izzie needed to acknowledge his betrayal, demonstrate that he was taking responsibility for it, and ask Amelia's forgiveness before considering working on the jealousy that might arise for both of them in a consensually open relationship.

JEALOUSY TRIGGERS

One of the most confusing things about jealousy is that while the *bodily sensations* of jealousy are very similar in everyone, varying mostly in intensity level, different people find that jealousy is triggered by different situations and different stimuli. In fact, some people feel that it's not useful or valid to lump all these different experiences together and call them by one name. I disagree.

In my experience coaching thousands of people on how to cope with their jealousy and in my own relationships, labeling all the many variations on how and why jealousy shows up as a single phenomenon does help people to handle this challenge more effectively. For one thing, this prevents people from disregarding jealous feelings until they get so intense that they become unmanageable, as we discussed earlier. For another, it helps people empathize with a partner's experience even when they do not share the same jealousy triggers. It also helps to short-circuit efforts to excuse or avoid taking responsibility for one's own jealousy by demanding that a partner change instead of negotiating coping strategies together.

However, it is definitely important to discover what is triggering a person's jealousy so that those involved can respond appropriately. Many people assume that the same things that make them jealous also make their partner(s) jealous. They then try to help by accommodating a loved one's vulnerability but can end up doing or saying precisely the wrong thing.

Peter suffered from feelings of inadequacy. He'd always had trouble believing that he was good enough to deserve the love and loyalty of his wife Sarah. When they agreed to open their marriage after ten years of harmonious domestic life, Peter was the first to get involved with someone else. He'd suspected that he was bisexual for a long time and finally took the risk of exploring an intimate relationship with another man. Sarah was supportive and relieved to find that she felt happy about Peter's having a new boyfriend. Then Peter, in a misguided effort to offer Sarah the reassurance that he would need if he were in her position, began telling Sarah that he didn't really think that highly of Mitchell (which wasn't true) and led her to believe that it was just a sexual attraction and certainly not love. Unfortunately, this had the exact opposite effect of what Peter intended. For Sarah, who was self-confident but proud, the thought that her husband was "sleeping around with just anyone" without any emotional involvement

wn center, cultivating other support systems, and fo-
nt moment rather than worrying about the past or the

lousy, fear of loss may also be present, but the primary
jealous person keeps comparing him- or herself with
otential lover and feels inadequate. The trigger is the
not good enough" or simply "I'm not enough," which is
ry that has been reactivated by present circumstances.
a partner won't leave doesn't help much to alleviate
of being undeserving of love since what the jealousy is
eed to see through the core story of not good enough.
he other lover can help dispel the illusion that he or she
etimes this type of jealousy can be easily managed by al
s person to create an "approved list" of nonthreatening
her partner to choose from.
s almost the polar opposite of competition jealousy. In this
the intensity of jealousy may increase instead of decrease if
s seen as unworthy or disagreeable in some way because the
is a concern about what others will think. If one's partner
ith a desirable lover, one can bask in the reflected glory, at
prous circles. Otherwise, a person with ego jealousy may not
y sharing a partner as long as no one else knows about the
afraid of being judged inadequate or powerless by others.
this type of jealousy is always the potential for being seen in
by others. The core of this type of jealousy is pride, and while
aged by negotiating appropriate agreements, its message is to
nd accept one's own vulnerability and cultivate humility.
Rick had enjoyed an open marriage for twelve years. During
h has had other relationships separately and sometimes dated
s well. Sophia is an attractive and confident woman who was
he'd never been jealous or possessive of Rick. She was much
this in the sexually open circles in which they'd always found
partners. When Rick began a relationship with a woman he'd
siness conference, Sophia experienced jealousy for the first
usiness associates are bound to notice," she complained. "They
what kind of relationship we have, that we've done this kind
years, and they just won't understand. I'm afraid they'll think
g on me."

was intolerable and quic
both. Peter's attempt to n
that Peter would become
they would judge her to be
ity was honorable, but casu

Dr. Ron Mazur, a forme
and categorized a range of
Intimacy. In brief, he distin
are described much more fu

All jealousy is not *possess*
sumed to be the case becaus
jealousy and the one most lik
acteristic attitude is, "I love y
than know you love someone
perceived threat to exclusive po
This type of jealousy is rarely an
is completely unwilling to consi
stances finds consensual nonmon

Possessive jealousy should not
common, although need not be pr
orous relationships. The concern h
Images of rejection, loneliness, and
fear of loss. The trigger for this typ
a partner *prefers* someone else, in c
attraction alone is the problem. In f
threatening if there is confidence tha
The unspoken assumption here is that
more likely and that falling in love wit
love with an existing partner. This may
not for others regardless of their identi
If fear jealousy is present, a deeply felt
will alleviate jealousy at least temporaril
from fear jealousy that their pain really
love interest, whether or not sex is invol
their beloved through death from a sudd
sage of fear jealousy is that you've come t
than on yourself for security and self-wor

time to feel one's o
cusing on the prese
future.

In *competition je*
problem is that the
another lover or p
thought that "I'm
usually an old sto
Reassurance that
internal feelings
revealing is the
Getting to know
is superior. Som
lowing the jealo
lovers for his or

Ego jealousy i
type of jealousy,
the other lover i
underlying issue
is connecting w
least in polyam
be disturbed b
situation but i
The trigger for
a negative ligh
it's easily man
learn to love a

Sophia and
this time, ea
as a couple a
proud that s
admired for
their other
met at a b
time. "His
don't know
of thing fo
he's cheati

was intolerable and quickly led to a jealous outburst that frightened them both. Peter's attempt to make Sarah more comfortable brought up her fear that Peter would become promiscuous, that others would find out, and that they would judge her to be promiscuous as well. In Sarah's mind, bisexuality was honorable, but casual sex was not.

Dr. Ron Mazur, a former minister and sex educator, has aptly named and categorized a range of different jealousy triggers in his book *The New Intimacy*. In brief, he distinguishes the following types of jealousy, which are described much more fully in his valuable resource.

All jealousy is not *possessive jealousy*, although this is sometimes assumed to be the case because this is the most dramatic manifestation of jealousy and the one most likely to lead to domestic violence. The characteristic attitude is, "I love you so much, I'd rather die or see you dead than know you love someone else." Possessive jealousy is triggered by a perceived threat to exclusive possession of the love object, that is, a spouse. This type of jealousy is rarely an issue in polyamory because someone who is completely unwilling to consider sharing a partner under any circumstances finds consensual nonmonogamy unthinkable.

Possessive jealousy should not be confused with *fear jealousy*, which is common, although need not be present, in both monogamous and polyamorous relationships. The concern here is loss of a partner to someone else. Images of rejection, loneliness, and scarcity usually accompany the primary fear of loss. The trigger for this type of jealousy can be any indication that a partner *prefers* someone else, in contrast to possessive jealousy, in which *attraction* alone is the problem. In fear jealousy, other attractions are not threatening if there is confidence that there's no threat of being replaced. The unspoken assumption here is that engaging in sex makes falling in love more likely and that falling in love with a new person means falling out of love with an existing partner. This may in fact be true for some people but not for others regardless of their identity as monogamous or polyamorous. If fear jealousy is present, a deeply felt renewal of trust and commitment will alleviate jealousy at least temporarily. I always remind people suffering from fear jealousy that their pain really has very little to do with the other love interest, whether or not sex is involved. They could just as easily lose their beloved through death from a sudden illness or accident. The message of fear jealousy is that you've come to depend more on your partner than on yourself for security and self-worth. It's best addressed by taking time to feel one's own center, cultivating other support systems, and focusing on the present moment rather than worrying about the past or the future.

In *competition jealousy*, fear of loss may also be present, but the primary problem is that the jealous person keeps comparing him- or herself with another lover or potential lover and feels inadequate. The trigger is the thought that "I'm not good enough" or simply "I'm not enough," which is usually an old story that has been reactivated by present circumstances. Reassurance that a partner won't leave doesn't help much to alleviate internal feelings of being undeserving of love since what the jealousy is revealing is the need to see through the core story of not good enough. Getting to know the other lover can help dispel the illusion that he or she is superior. Sometimes this type of jealousy can be easily managed by allowing the jealous person to create an "approved list" of nonthreatening lovers for his or her partner to choose from.

Ego jealousy is almost the polar opposite of competition jealousy. In this type of jealousy, the intensity of jealousy may increase instead of decrease if the other lover is seen as unworthy or disagreeable in some way because the underlying issue is a concern about what others will think. If one's partner is connecting with a desirable lover, one can bask in the reflected glory, at least in polyamorous circles. Otherwise, a person with ego jealousy may not be disturbed by sharing a partner as long as no one else knows about the situation but is afraid of being judged inadequate or powerless by others. The trigger for this type of jealousy is always the potential for being seen in a negative light by others. The core of this type of jealousy is pride, and while it's easily managed by negotiating appropriate agreements, its message is to learn to love and accept one's own vulnerability and cultivate humility.

Sophia and Rick had enjoyed an open marriage for twelve years. During this time, each has had other relationships separately and sometimes dated as a couple as well. Sophia is an attractive and confident woman who was proud that she'd never been jealous or possessive of Rick. She was much admired for this in the sexually open circles in which they'd always found their other partners. When Rick began a relationship with a woman he'd met at a business conference, Sophia experienced jealousy for the first time. "His business associates are bound to notice," she complained. "They don't know what kind of relationship we have, that we've done this kind of thing for years, and they just won't understand. I'm afraid they'll think he's cheating on me."

8

Exclusion jealousy, which is sometimes also called *time jealousy*, is very common in polyamory. Like ego jealousy, people often resist identifying this variation as a form of jealousy, but the bodily sensations and behaviors are often indistinguishable from other types of jealousy. The issue is not reluctance to share a partner but rather fear that others are not going to share with you in turn. Sometimes there is a desire to be included at all times instead of having separate dates. Exclusion jealousy is triggered when the jealous person feels that he or she is being left out of the fun or deprived of equal time and attention. This kind of jealousy can be especially intense when a new and exciting lover has recently arrived, and the perception of neglect is real. When this is the case, I coach people to remember that "new relationship energy" is temporary but intoxicating. A partner can easily get carried away by new relationship energy but eventually will come to his or her senses. A long-term partner has a history of commitment and loyalty that no newcomer can match, while any new love can get those euphoric neurotransmitters pumping. It takes some maturity and willingness to surrender control, but that's what this form of jealousy is asking of us. Sometimes time jealousy can be managed by scheduling "date nights" when all partners see outside lovers at the same time or by prioritizing quality time with an existing partner before seeing others.

JEALOUSY AND THE PARENTAL TRIANGLE

Glamorous Rachael had recently left a ten-year open marriage with Henry, an older man who was a popular workshop leader and therapist. She approached Bev and Gene about developing an intimate relationship with them and went out of her way to cultivate a friendship with Bev before requesting permission for a sexual encounter with Gene. Bev and Gene had been lovers for five years. They were strongly bonded with an agreement that each could include others sexually. Bev and Gene chose not to live together, partly to facilitate their open relationship. When Rachael suggested that they all have a three-way date the following week, Bev readily agreed. On the afternoon of their date, Rachael stopped by to visit Gene and ended up having sex with him and coaxing an ejaculation from Gene, who had a strong preference for nonejaculatory orgasms. When Rachael and Gene showed up at Bev's home for the planned date, Gene was feeling withdrawn and sexually depleted and suggested that they go to a movie instead of making love as planned. Bev tried to be accepting and understanding, but jealousy overtook her, and she had a "hissy fit," as she put it. When she later consulted me for help in "curing" her unanticipated jealous reaction, she was confused and bewildered. "I can't understand it," she sobbed. "I thought Rachael was my friend, and I was excited about getting closer to her. Gene wasn't that enthusiastic about her at first, but now he doesn't want to agree to stop seeing her."

A woman who tends to be competitive with other women often had a mother who didn't support her feminine expression. Both mother and daughter are insecure in their own power as women. This kind of mother may have been jealous of her husband's attention to the daughter or fearful of incest because of her own background and try to come in between them. She's threatened by her daughter's innocent childlike sexuality and may punish it because she feels uncomfortable with and cut off from her own sexuality. A woman who had a mother like this must try very hard to appear feminine and sexy to make up for her inner doubts. She's often seductive and flirtatious but doesn't really want the man once she has him. She tends to play a submissive role with a dominant man whom she ends up resenting and fearing. She desperately needs the support of other women but has trouble getting it because she's always competing with women to win the prize of male attention.

When this type of woman is unaware of her inner dynamics, she often imagines that she wants a relationship with an established couple. Consciously, she may be seeking a close relationship with a woman who will be the supportive "good mother" and role model she didn't find with her own mother and who will protect her from becoming lost in the man's orbit. Unconsciously, her agenda is to reenact her childhood drama and to take Daddy away from Mommy. Sometimes the woman in the couple will sense this and become inexplicably jealous. If she overrides her intuition, she may find that the newcomer who seemed so agreeable has seduced her partner away while refusing any intimacy with her. Meanwhile, the interloper justifies distancing from the coupled woman on the grounds that she's too angry and emotionally unsafe.

A man whose father was insecure in his masculinity and was constantly trying to prove his worth by competing with other males, including his son, also tends to have a difficult time with same-gender cooperation in polyamorous relationships. This type of man, who can often be described as dominant, alpha, or macho, enjoys having a harem of adoring women but has trouble sharing their affections with other men. Like his father before him, the son didn't get the male support he desperately needed because his father viewed him as a threat to be battled for the love and attention of the boy's mother. As an adult, if he hasn't consciously transformed his childhood patterns, he will deny that he's jealous while unconsciously competing with any man his partner tries to introduce into their relationship. He will often deny any responsibility for driving prospective partners away and project his competitiveness onto the other man. The scenario of the other man whose agenda is to "cut that little filly out of the herd" is also a common one in men with unresolved father issues. His target can be either a monogamous or an open couple or a powerful man who has acquired more than one woman. He often loses interest in the woman once he's wooed her away from her partner.

The intoxication of a new romantic relationship can easily override the discernment of those involved. Consequently, in an open relationship, cues may be missed by the individual with a new lover but show up loud and clear to an established partner who is then accused of jealousy and possessiveness when they share their fears. For this reason—and many others, as we discuss in the next sections—those who hope for successful polyamorous relationships would do well to clear up their family-of-origin issues before they begin.

COMPERSION

Compersion is a word created by the Kerista Community to describe an emotion that is the opposite of jealousy. Compersion means to feel joy and delight when one's beloved loves or is being loved by another. Compersion is especially strong and accessible when all the people involved have feelings of love for each other, but that's not a necessary precondition.

Some people have spontaneously had the experience of compersion, much to their surprise, when they were anticipating feeling jealous. Some find compersion as natural and inevitable as jealousy seems to be for others. People like this instantly recognize their feeling as compersion as soon as they hear the new term.

However, since most of us have been raised with an expectation of jealousy, compersion is an alien concept. Learning theory tells us that it's always easier to replace one habit with another than to just eliminate the first one. If you can't imagine feeling compersion instead of jealousy, you can try the following experiment the next time you feel jealous. Instead of focusing on your own discomfort and fears, try putting your attention on your partner. Think of the happiness and pleasure your partner may be experiencing and how your partner's good feelings will eventually be passed on to you. If this seems impossible, try imagining a situation which is less threatening to you but still touches on your jealousy triggers.

Just having a concept that acknowledges that you have an alternative to feeling jealous can go a long way toward transforming jealousy. It really is possible to feel joy and expansion rather than fear and contraction in response to a loved one's sharing their love with others, as thousands of people can attest. But it's not always easy. My e-book *Compersion: Using Jealousy as a Path to Unconditional Love* offers ways to reprogram your thinking away from jealousy and toward compersion while bringing the valuable messages jealousy brings into awareness.

Jealousy has a spiritual dimension. In essence, jealousy indicates a crisis of faith. It is part of conditional love. If you will love only when you're assured of having your love returned, then you make yourself vulnerable to jealousy. On a more practical level, we could say simply that jealousy is a sign that your relationship needs work of some kind. For example, jealousy can be a message that your relation *is* changing. Rather than fearing the changes and struggling against them, jealousy can instead be a message to surrender to change and trust that if you set her free, she'll return if she truly belongs with you. Or jealousy could be bringing your attention to your own fear of abandonment, showing you that if you fail to address the source of this fear in you, you may indeed drive your partner away.

In order to make the most of jealousy as an opportunity for growth, I always coach people to discharge or manage the intensity of the emotional reaction itself so that jealousy's teachings can be received. Sometimes all that's needed is to wait for a more suitable time to confront jealousy head-on rather than foolishly rushing in where angels fear to tread. If your bodymind is swamped with overwhelmingly chaotic sensations, you're in no position to learn anything.

MANAGING JEALOUSY

I always encourage people to find an appropriate balance between becoming skillful at finding ways to sidestep jealousy and avoid the turmoil it brings and inviting jealousy to become a powerful teacher who can show us the places we most need healing and motivate us to grow beyond our perceived limits so that we're capable of more love. Part of the difficulty in managing jealousy is that most people have gotten conflicting messages about it. One the one hand, it's inevitable and part of love. On the other, it's shameful and a sign of weakness. Hence, working with jealousy always entails working with the shadow. When people manage their jealousy too well, they limit their own potential or may find themselves adapting to a disempowering situation.

The first step in managing jealousy is admitting to yourself and your partner(s) that it's a problem. When people try to keep a stiff upper lip and deny that they're jealous, they usually sabotage themselves by allowing their jealousy to build until it really is unmanageable. It's far better to acknowledge the first stirrings of jealousy and learn to listen respectfully to the part of yourself that feels jealous without believing everything you hear. If this isn't a process you're familiar with, seek the help of an experienced therapist until disidentifying with your emotions and dialoguing with conflicting parts become second nature. Most people tend to leap prematurely into action to change the situation instead of pausing a moment to integrate this uncomfortable experience and reclaim their shadow self.

Asking for support from friends as well as partners is an important way to take care of yourself even when you're familiar with navigating these turbulent emotional currents. Communicating as clearly as you can what you're experiencing and making specific requests without engaging in blame or making demands can be amazingly effective.

Chuck noticed a churning sensation in his gut when he saw his girlfriend Janice holding hands with Frank and looking adoringly into his eyes. As soon as Janice and Frank disengaged, he asked Janice if she could spend a few minutes with him. "I notice that I'm feeling separate from you," he said, "and I don't want to feel that way. Can we hold each other so I can connect with you again?" Janice quickly agreed, happy that Chuck wasn't blaming her for his upset, relieved that his request was so easy to fulfill, and genuinely appreciating and loving him more than ever.

Not everyone is as self-aware and skillful at communicating and letting go as Chuck. Just taking some deep breaths, vigorous exercise, yoga, dance, massage, listening to relaxing music, a breathwork session, or even watching a funny or uplifting movie are all good ways to dissipate the charge of jealousy *before* thinking about or discussing the specifics of the situation that triggered the jealousy. Trying to have a rational and reasonable conversation with a jealous person is useless at best and very likely counterproductive.

Once the emotional storm has passed or before it has blown in is a far better time to work on identifying your personal jealousy triggers and ask your partner to help find ways to work around them. Many partners will resist taking total responsibility for managing another's jealousy but are usually happy to negotiate solutions that help each get what they want. The key is to approach managing jealousy as a shared project both can cooperate on instead of pitting one person against another or allowing one partner to use his or her jealousy to manipulate the other or make the other wrong.

If one partner is resistant to teamwork, it's worth investigating whether there's a payoff in having a jealous partner. For example, Joseph refused to empathize with Suzy's jealous reaction when he ignored her all evening and focused his attention on Jill, whom he'd met for the first time at the dinner party all three were attending. When they came to me for help with Suzy's jealousy, Joseph rejected Suzy's request that he give her equal time and express more appreciation, saying that she was trying to control him. It soon became apparent that Joseph enjoyed triggering Suzy's jealousy. They were in the midst of a power struggle, and bringing out Suzy's insecurity and fear of abandonment tipped the scales in his favor. Other people may prefer a partner who is more jealous than they are or who they are not fully attracted to so that they never have to confront their own insecurity or vulnerability. These kinds of dynamics need to be resolved before jealousy can be successfully managed.

When there are no obstacles in the way and both people are genuinely interesting in helping each other get what they want, negotiation can go a long way toward reducing jealousy to manageable levels. Elizabeth and Tom discussed polyamory on their first date and were delighted to find that neither one of them was interested in monogamy. But after their marriage a year later, Elizabeth found herself feeling possessive. When Candace flirted with Tom at a party, Elizabeth felt the first stirrings of jealousy. Still, she accepted when Candace invited her to lunch, and when Candace asked her permission to have a date with Tom, Elizabeth found her jealousy nearly disappearing. Realizing that being asked for permission made a big difference in her comfort level, Elizabeth asked Tom to instruct any woman he wanted to date to ask Elizabeth's permission first. Tom was happy to find such a simple means to manage Elizabeth's jealousy and conscientiously complied with her request. "There's only been one woman Elizabeth said 'no' to in the past three years and one who refused to ask her, out of six women I've been interested in. I'm a lucky man!"

Neil's jealousy was not so easily dealt with. When Neil and Lynne decided to embark on an open relationship after four years of marriage, he found that while he valued the freedom to enjoy intimacy with other women, he couldn't stand the prospect of Lynne making love with another man who she might like better than him. Neil asked Lynne to agree that they get involved only with married couples since he felt safer with men who were already in a committed relationship. Lynne was willing to try this for one year if Neil would agree to work on his jealousy during that time and renegotiate at the end of the year.

I suggested that Neil use systematic desensitization to reduce his emotional reactivity enough to investigate the source of his jealousy. Together we constructed a detailed list of scenarios that triggered jealousy for him, ordered from the least threatening to the most threatening. With Lynne's support, he chose a time when they were feeling relaxed and comfortable with each other to try imagining the least difficult scene, which for him was a double date with another couple. Neil was able to stay relaxed and free of jealousy until he began visualizing that after dinner and dancing, the two couples returned to their home and Lynne went into their bedroom with the other man, leaving Neil in the living room with the other woman. He'd gone too far too fast and needed to take smaller steps.

The following week, Neil tried again, changing the scenario so that both couples went into the bedroom and made love side by side with their own partners and then all engaged in "pillow talk" together. This time Neil felt only a small twinge of jealousy. Gradually over several sessions, he adjusted his fantasy to increase the amount of contact Lynne had with the other man. Then he tried imagining Lynne and the other man getting out of bed and going into the living room, leaving Neil alone with the other woman. This scenario felt so comfortable that Neil decided to give his original fantasy of Lynne going into their bedroom with the other man after a double date another try. Once again his jealousy overwhelmed him.

I advised Neil to try imagining another location, such as a two-room suite in a hotel. The hotel scenario worked much better for him. Neil was able to picture Lynne spending the rest of the night with the other man in their hotel suite without feeling much jealousy at all. Neil had unknowingly hit one of his own jealousy buttons by thinking about Lynne in their own special bed with another man.

Some months later, Neil and Lynne met a couple both of them liked and were able to develop a warm friendship that slowly became sexual after Neil shared his struggle with jealousy and asked to rendezvous at a hotel. Neil remained jealousy free until Lynne told him she wanted to go away for the weekend with the other man. He again implemented the systematic desensitization technique and after several weeks of work felt he was ready to send Lynne off for the weekend. I coached him to plan some activities for himself during this time, and he decided to take advantage of the opportunity to go river rafting, which was not something Lynne enjoyed. When Lynne asked if *he* would go away with her the following weekend, Neil knew his hard work had paid off, and he eagerly asked me for some instruction on how to let jealousy be his teacher.

Systematic desensitization is a useful technique but it doesn't always work to manage jealousy, especially if the jealousy is intense and the ability to negotiate agreements to avoid the biggest triggers is absent for one reason or another. For some people, in some situations, jealousy does seem to dictate ending a valued relationship.

Patricia and Bruce met at a polyamory conference and soon fell in love. Their respective spouses were supportive until Bruce's jealousy became a problem. Bruce wasn't jealous of Patricia's husband in the least. "I love my wife," Bruce explained, "and I want to stay married to her. I'm glad that Patricia has a good relationship with Ellis too. I just can't stand the thought of her meeting another guy who might take my place. She says two great men are enough for her, and she's not looking for anyone else, but Ellis wants her to go to parties and on dinner dates with other couples so *he* can meet someone. She's a very social person and enjoys hanging out with all her poly friends. Even if Ellis was willing to meet women without her, I don't think it's fair to ask her to give up all her friends. Besides, she wouldn't do it anyway."

Patricia and Ellis were willing to temporarily alter their social life while Bruce tried to reduce the intensity of his jealousy and get to the source of his jealous fear. He had some success, but as soon as Patricia and Ellis returned to their usual way of life, Bruce's jealousy became unbearable. "It's strange," Bruce said miserably, "I'm not at all jealous with my wife Zoë, but I just can't get over it with Patricia. Some relationships are just different. I can't do this any more! It's just too hard." Bruce had made a valiant effort, but in the end jealousy had its way with him.

7

POLYAMORY AND CHILDREN

Many people assume that it's harmful for children to have more than two parents. Of course, multiple parents are common in stepfamilies, where a child may have as many as four parents from two blended families. In the many cultures where polygyny is permitted, children often grow up with several mothers who cooperate in caring for each other's children. And from time immemorial, older brothers and sisters, as well as extended families of grandparents, aunts, uncles, and cousins, have shared family compounds and taken on significant roles as caretakers. One of the most indelible images from all my travels is a slender elderly man with a wizened face squatting beside a toddler just after dawn in the outskirts of a village in central India. This man looked at the little one, who I imagined to be his grandchild, with a look of such love and devotion that I literally stopped in my tracks, unable to shift my gaze.

As extended families who live together become increasingly rare, especially in the affluent West, polyamorous families are one way that some people are counteracting the isolation of the lone nuclear family and finding ways to provide at-home caretakers for children. Others gravitate toward cohousing or intentional communities that may or may not be monogamously oriented but where adults share some responsibility for child rearing.

Several studies have been done on stepfamilies and children reared communally, but there is still a dearth of research investigating the important question of how polyamory affects children. At the same time, the impact on children is one of the most commonly asked questions whenever the subject of polyamory is raised. Dr. Elisabeth Sheff is an assistant professor of sociology at Georgia State University. She conducted her doctoral research on polyamorous families with children in the mid-1990s and later decided to attempt a longitudinal study of these and other poly families. So far, she's following about thirty families with three or more adults living together who have children between the ages of six and twenty. She'd like to double that and include an ethnically and culturally more diversified group before publishing her findings but says that funding for research on polyamory is scarce.

Dr. Sheff's research focuses on families where three or more adults in committed relationships jointly share responsibility for child rearing. However, open marriages are far more common than group marriages and consequently are impacting many more children. Single parents with intimate networks also are increasingly common and present a similar milieu for children in many respects. All these types of multipartner relationships may shape children's experiences in a variety of ways that have not even begun to be considered, except by theorists and the parents themselves, let alone researched.

As a parent who has raised two children of my own in a variety of non-monogamous contexts and watched many friends and clients do the same over the years, I have thought deeply about these issues and written several articles on the subject. As I began to undertake the writing of this book, I interviewed at least one parent and sometimes children in fifteen different families where one or more children lived with a nonmonogamous parent, most often in open marriages. The youngest child is currently one year old, and many of the children are now young adults in their early twenties who are engaged in their own intimate relationships. In addition, over the years, I've socialized with, coached, or spoken at length with at least several hundred other polyamorous families with children and a few dozen middle-aged adults who were raised in families where their parents had open or group marriages or where patriarchal-style polygamy was practiced.

In an open marriage or single-parent household, it's quite common for secondary partners to visit regularly, stay over on weekends, or stay for weeks at a time and perhaps for them to become housemates or to move in for a trial period as a prelude to a more permanent arrangement. In situations like this, lovers often take on roles similar to those of aunts and uncles rather than coparents. Parents must decide how and when to integrate these visitors into the family and what, if anything, to say to the children about the new lover who is now sharing Mommy and/or Daddy's bed.

All the recent surveys of polyamorous people find that about half of them are parents (see chapter 2 for details on demographics). However, at least half of these attempt to hide their extramarital relationships from their children or have teens or adult children whose lives are mainly independent of their parents or utilize polyamorous gatherings, other social occasions, or coaching sessions as a vacation from parenting. As a result, in the course of everyday life, I've had far less opportunity to interact with the children of polys than with their parents, except in the case of personal friends where spending time with the entire family was a natural part of our interactions. Consequently, while I believe my observations can be generalized to a wider population, this may not be the case. It's possible that the children of poly parents I have not met are different from those that I have met. I've attempted to remedy this by including representative interviews that allow the reader to get a feel for the person who is talking and draw their own conclusions.

In addition, Dr. Sheff agreed to share the preliminary findings from her research with me. Her sample is also skewed in that virtually all her participants thus far come from the network of people who strongly identify as polyamorous and who attend various polyamorous conferences, potluck dinners, or other social events. Dr. Sheff has found that some polyamorous parents are reluctant to talk to anyone "official" because they are concerned about losing custody of their children. The common perception that children in poly (and nonheterosexual) families are at higher risk for sexual abuse than those in monogamous families, which appears to be completely unfounded according to Dr. Sheff, also makes people nervous about talking to her. Her focus has been to rely on unstructured interviews to determine what kinds of experiences children in polyamorous families have, what the internal dynamics of the family are, and what kinds of things these families do that help them survive. Further, she's included nonbiological parents who she says are sometimes more involved in the day-to-day parenting than the biological parents, perhaps because they have more time and inclination for it. Nevertheless, as I spoke with my own contacts and heard what she had found thus far, a cohesive picture began to emerge.

In the absence of existing research on polyamorous families, Dr. Sheff has looked to the research on children of gays and lesbians for clues. There's a fair amount of this research, she says, because much of it is funded from within the gay and lesbian communities themselves who have a "we are family" campaign that funds research as well as political activity. The lion's share of sexuality research money is also going to the study of gay, lesbian, bisexual, and transgendered (GLBT) issues, and the little funding that exists for family research comes mostly from conservative groups for whom polyamory is not of interest. The GLBT research has found that essentially all the pressure the children of homosexual parents face is from outside the family. In other words, nothing has been found in the families themselves that's a problem for the children, but they do encounter judgments, prejudice, and negative attitudes from outsiders, such as teachers or neighbors, or are concerned about appearing different. The same appears to be somewhat true for children in polyamorous families, although one bisexual poly parent told me that his teenage son's perception was that polyamory was more acceptable than bisexuality among his peers.

Geography, as well as individual differences, no doubt plays a role in the extent to which children of polyamorous families encounter prejudice or feel different. I've been told by people in Europe and Australia that this is definitely an issue, while for many of the children in Dr. Sheff's study who live in the San Francisco Bay Area, it's not. Dr. Samuel Widmer is a Swiss psychiatrist who has five school-age children with his partner Daniele and another four children between ages three and eleven with his other partner Marianne. He reports that they all live together happily and think nothing of it until they start school. "Afterwards, they go through different stages of looking at it. But all of them so far always again find a positive outlook. They are proud to be special."[1]

Australian researcher and educator Dr. Maria Pallotta-Chiarolli points to the need for addressing the ways in which children in polyamorous families may experience discrimination, prejudice, and misunderstanding both from "the wider heteronormative society and from within the gay and lesbian community."[2] One anecdote about two aboriginal boys is illuminating. While these students are likely even more sensitive to possible repercussions than white Australians, I could imagine similar scenarios among American minorities as well.

"The two students were not 'cousins' as they labelled themselves at school: that was the word they used for whites to prevent suspicion. Their mothers were not blood-sisters but certainly sisters. They shared the same husband, the children shared the same father. They all lived happily in one house. At school, the children kept to themselves in order to discourage any intimacy with other children that could lead to discovery and a further reason to harass them as they were already experiencing ongoing racist harassment. They had also been warned by their parents not to let white teachers know or else they'd be taken away from their family, a theme that was all too real for this family whose own childhoods had been mostly spent in mission homes after being removed from their families as part of Australia's racist assimilationist policies."[3]

Australian whites also reported problems in the schools. Two blood sisters who share the same husband and are raising their children together reported that "it's been harder with the school and for now, the less said to them the better. We worry they may get some child welfare person who may decide this is an unfit or dysfunctional home just based on the fact that we're poly. Or if one of the kids got into trouble at school, there used to be this assumption that it had to do with their home background. Slowly, that's blown over as the kids are happy and healthy. But they've also experienced some teasing from other kids and they tend to be careful who they say things to. It's not fair that kids should have to worry about such things."[4]

Dr. Pallotta-Chiarolli decided that writing a novel for young adults would be one way to support teens who are struggling to reconcile the realities of their bisexual and/or polyamorous families with the heteronormative mainstream culture. The result was *Love You Two*,[5] which is the tale of Pina, a young Australian woman who accidentally discovers that her mother loves two men. Then, when she turns to her uncle for help, she learns that he's bisexual. It's all very confusing for Pina, who loves her mother but has trouble integrating the realization that there are different ways to love.

Dr. Sheff reports that in the United States, the majority of the children she's talked to have been pretty relaxed about their parents' relationship orientation. Most say that it's fine with them, that they have no problems with it, or that the advantages outweigh the disadvantages, but this might not be the case in families who are less openly polyamorous or live in more conservative areas. Some of the advantages mentioned are that they get more attention, more help with homework, and more people to give them rides. They have other adults to go to if they have a problem they don't want to take to their parents. Sheff found that the poly family is often a resource for tween and teen friends of the family for sex education. They tend to be comfortable with and available for discussing sexual issues and are a source of reliable information—*not* having sex in front of them or with them, Dr. Sheff stresses. In contrast to the findings in the gay and lesbian families and in Australia, only one boy in her sample said that it's been bad for him because he feels he can't bring friends home without having to explain it all, so it hurts his social life. Others commented on it being painful when a parent's partner who they've gotten attached to leaves, but of course this is sometimes a problem in monogamous families who divorce especially when the noncustodial parent doesn't maintain contact or has an acrimonious relationship with the ex-spouse.

The only other research that I'm aware of in the United States that looked at children in group marriages was a study done by Larry and Joan Constantine in the 1970s, but they did not investigate the children's interface with schools or the wider society in which they lived. The Constantines conducted their research on a self-funded shoestring, outside of academia, and while they used psychological measures and other objective data in addition to personal interviews, they were admittedly biased in favor of what they then called *multilateral marriage*. Nevertheless, they reported that the children in these multiadult families were, on the whole, far above average in terms of self-esteem, academic performance, and social skills.[6]

I asked Dr. Sheff whether she saw the older children choosing polyamory for themselves, and she said that mostly they were still too young to have really made a choice, but it seems to vary. One nineteen-year-old boy said, "Why would I want to limit myself when I'm so young? It's natural to be attracted to more than one girl." A teenage girl said, "No way! I need too much attention and I'm too jealous for polyamory. I can't imagine how my mother has done it all these years!"[7] Is the traditional gender divide showing itself in the next generation? Two data points are not enough to draw any conclusions, but perhaps one day Dr. Sheff's research will help answer this question and others. Meanwhile, my conversation with Raymond may shed some light on the relational choices of the next generation.

THE NEXT GENERATION

Raymond is the twenty-year-old son of my friend Becca. I first met him when he was a young teen and was immediately impressed by his poise, warmth, and good humor as he greeted me and welcomed me into their home. Unlike many teens who tend to treat adults with suspicion or disdain, he animatedly took part in the dinner conversation, which spanned a number of complex social and ecological issues, and offered to loan me a paper he'd written for a school project on one of the topics we'd been discussing. Raymond is a handsome and athletic young man, as comfortable in his body and with his emotions as he is with words and ideas. He's now a college student with a steady girlfriend.

Raymond spent his early years in Puerto Rico in a happy family that consisted of his mother and father, Will, and his mother's girlfriend Marta. The sexual relationship between the two women eventually expanded to include Will. All three enjoyed working and playing together as well as nurturing Raymond. After a few years, Marta got involved with another man who became her primary partner, but they all remained close friends. Some years after that, Becca and Will split up, and Becca eventually linked up with JG and moved to Italy, then returned to the United States for Raymond's high school years. Her description of the care with which she introduced JG into the household is characteristic of her sensitive and protective stance toward Raymond, even as she embarked on a sexually open, polyamorous life.

"Raising kids in an 'alternative lifestyle' household can be tricky," Becca admits, "not so much because of the kids part but because of the alternative part. I always respected Raymond's integrity as a person. So that meant that in our house, stability, acceptance, and communication were top values. If a new relationship was developing, this new person would become a frequent dinner guest or visitor but not to the point of disturbing the family rhythm. When JG and I were seeing each other is a case in point, even though this was not a polyamorous situation at the time; we were just getting together as a couple. Since this was my first serious relationship after leaving my sixteen-year relationship with Raymond's father, I was hypersensitive about disruption in my son's life, so I only allowed JG to spend the night on weekends, when Raymond was at his dad's house. Finally, after nearly nine months, Raymond was going to be with us the whole weekend, and he pleaded, 'Can't JG do a sleepover? Can't he spend the night tonight?' Raymond felt so comfortable with JG that he considered him *his* buddy (which JG had for some time been pointing out to me). From then on, we relaxed more into family mode.

"When other lovers then entered into our sphere, I kept the sexual encounters out of Raymond's view. As far as he was concerned, these were new friends who were hanging around, and he was certainly benefiting from the new perspectives around the dinner table and fun outings with interesting people. It's not that I think sex is something to be hidden, but maturing into one's sexuality is a process, with experience that is age appropriate to each stage. Polyamory is alternative, and in some places that is threatening. We had a friend whose neighbor called Social Services because she was letting her preschoolers run around the yard naked. Then for months this mother had to deal with surprise visits from social workers. We could not risk such visits because on the walls of our house hung erotic art—explicitly erotic art that formed part of the book we were working on: *The Pillow Book of Venus and Her Lover—Reinventing the Myth*.[8] It was a dynamic in our household, too, because James regularly showed up from his art studio with a new painting, which we celebrated. Then I would write a poem to the painting and debut it in front of James and Raymond.

"In the early years, I did not want to expose Raymond to the art because I felt he was too young to understand it, but as a tween, he began posing his first sexual questions, so we used the paintings to illustrate our answers. And our answers were from a Tantric perspective: That love between/among people was the greatest human experience, that not only could the power of love awaken a person's potential as a human being but also a person's spiritual magnificence. So the 'sex talk' with my son was more like a roundtable discussion among the three of us that lasted years.

"From our relaxed openness, Raymond got the impression there was nothing wrong with sexual love, and this is more important than whatever details he might have known or not known about our sex lives. The atmosphere in our home was one of inclusiveness, candor, creativity, cooperation, and comaraderie. We did have to keep reminding him that repression out in the world also existed. We told him he had to keep the paintings and our other lovers a secret because we did not want Social Services knocking on our door or threatening to take him away from us. I was raised in a sexually repressed family where sex was only for procreation, as far as my siblings and I could tell. It was my intention to end that family tradition with my son.

"Raymond didn't have the fear or shame around sex that his friends had picked up in their families. Still, when he got to high school, he had a girlfriend who was jealous, and he also fell into the jealousy trap. Since it had never been part of our world, I was surprised to see him go through jealousy. But then, Raymond was his own person and had to go through the lessons himself. Because of our openness, however, he had the advantage of still coming to us with his struggles, so we could help him find his way."

When I asked Becca how she thought her polyamorous lifestyle had affected her son, she said, "I hear of the ups and downs of his relationships, just like any normal young man. So while I would like to say that our sexualoving lifestyle saved him such grief, I see that is not so. On the other hand, he sees the slings and arrows of his love life as part of his spiritual path, and I also notice that he truly honors his girlfriends and maintains friendships with old lovers. As a mother, then, I do not worry about him. He has the tools necessary to navigate his course through life. I am not the only one who thinks so, either; when he graduated from high school, he was awarded the annual scholarship given to the one student 'who represented the greatest hope for the world.' What the scholarship committee may or may not have realized—but what I know—is that by being raised in a nonrepressive environment, Raymond was allowed to develop his whole self, which includes his intellectual, spiritual, physical, and sexual identities."

Raymond himself openly discusses his relationship history in an amazingly insightful way for a young man. "When I was fifteen, I was very interested in a girl but refused to get into a relationship with her because, for one thing, she lived hours away, and she wanted me to commit to only her. I didn't want an exclusive relationship. I would've reacted differently now, however, because there was no one else I was actually interested in at the time. So why not have a relationship with her? But I thought I might meet someone else. I wanted freedom, without taking enough responsibility. Now I take my current girlfriend's feelings more into account, even if I don't agree with them. Back then I had a mental, rational thing of not wanting to be monogamous because of who I am and who my parents are. I was being in my head instead of feeling it out, but I didn't realize—I don't have a need to *not* be in monogamous relationship now. Why not make a commitment with her?

"I had close relationships with other girls at the time because of how it was with those girls. A group of us surfed together, went on camping trips together, but while we touched and hugged a lot, it wasn't really sexual. We enjoyed hanging around each other. My two closest female friends were attractive to me, but we had a deeper friendship. Now at college, girls will act like they're hitting on you, but they're just being loving with you. Sometimes it's confusing.

"Living in the *Venus and Her Lover* household did contribute to the maturing of my sexual identity. I was more mature than most kids without going through that interior shit. So first I learned this framework on how to go about my relationships . . . a higher vision. It was a positive thing in my life. It gave me something to look towards. Then I started having a girlfriend, and there was my own interior personal stuff working that out in relationships. Okay, Mom and JG act this way, but what does it really mean? Cool ideas, now let me internalize that. Then, I've had to work through it all on my own.

"I had the same girlfriend my junior and senior years in high school. We studied together, we were on the swim team together, we had fun together. But she was very jealous, I would get jealous, and we would argue . . . drama. Yes, I was horny and wanting to have sex, but even more, I thought: I've learned a lot about a healthy functional relationship, but I've never experienced a dysfunctional relationship. I did have a love for her, and I thought: even though I'm unhappy with how things are, I'm learning so much. I just need to go through it. It taught me a lot of what I didn't want, on a deeper level, not just in my head from what I learned from my parents. Being able to talk to your parents about your relationships and sexuality is a big advantage! It cuts out a whole ton of shit. It provides more clarity on those very personal questions. If you can only seek answers from society and friends, they can give you a skewed view of life.

"I feel blessed that I've been exposed to more conscious relationship. Now that I'm in relationships it's helping me now more than when I was a kid. I will say that something I've been realizing more is that the whole idea of a free and open relationship, when I was in high school, was totally cool and groovy, but at my maturity level then, I took that free, open relationship idea as more like a selfish, egocentric thing. I thought I could do more of what I wanted, if I hurt my girlfriend, then that's her problem, she's jealous. Since then, I've reflected more on it, and now with my girlfriend, I have more of an understanding for other people's feelings, so I understand how other people feel about it. I can see a value in monogamy. I would have to work it out if I chose polyamory. To have an open relationship, there needs to be a greater level of maturity. Interior work that needs to happen before polyamory, and then you have to really work at it. I didn't notice any of that before because my parents made it seem so easy and normal." What parent wouldn't be proud to have raised a young man like this one.

Nora and Jim are also proud of their two children: Adam, who is now twenty-four, and Carla, who is twenty-one. Adam is completing his doctorate in biochemistry and has been dating his current girlfriend for about a year, Carla recently finished college and is living with her girlfriend in a monogamous relationship. Nora describes the children as "happy campers" and is close to both. At first glance, they're a conventional, normal-looking family. But Nora says their lesbian daughter is the most conservative of the lot.

Nora and Jim began dating thirty-five years ago and have been married for almost thirty years. Both were virgins when they got together in high school but agreed to explore sexually with others while they were away at different colleges, knowing that they would marry one day. He's now a successful attorney, and she's a psychotherapist in the New York suburbs. Fifteen years ago, after twenty years of monogamy, Nora and Jim embarked on an intimate relationship with the parents of Carla's best friend. Carla was in kindergarten at the time. Nora recalls that they started to talk openly to the children about their polyamorous lifestyle a few years later because they felt it was important for them to know what was going on in the family. At the time, the children were too young to be asking questions about the sexual arrangements, but they wanted Adam and Carla to know that these extra adults who were spending so much time in their home were people their parents loved and cared about.

Nora says that the relationship with this first couple, which was initiated by the other woman who said that she "liked what you have" and wanted help bolstering her own floundering marriage, ended when the other couple got divorced. "We probably helped them stay together a little longer, but in the end we couldn't rescue them," Nora explains. But it was the beginning of a new chapter in her own marriage. For the next eight years, Nora lived with first one and then another lover in the family home while Jim had long-term relationships with two women sequentially who would spend most weekends at their house. Son Adam took it all in stride but now says, "I had no clue why you were hanging out with these baby-men, Mom." Carla was a little less sanguine, especially as a teenager. She didn't like having extra adults living in her house and once asked her mother, "Why can't you be normal and get divorced like everyone else?" In retrospect, Nora regrets that their intense relationships with people who were single and sometimes "needy" took time and energy away from the children but feels that the children also benefited from relating to more adults. "They each have lots of friends, are very social and have excellent communication skills, way above average," she says.

The biggest challenge came when Nora and Jim, along with their respective lovers, agreed to be profiled in a national magazine. Jim's family got very upset about the publicity, and it created a lot of tension, especially with his sister who had been very close to the children and completely withdrew for a while. "It all blew over after a year or so," Nora says. "It was kind of ridiculous, she knew our partners, they'd been at her wedding, but that's how families are sometimes."

Jacob also has two children in their early twenties. Jacob and his ex-wife Karen had an open marriage before their two girls were born, but he found that running his business along with providing the best possible environment for the children took too much time and energy to continue pursuing other relationships. Karen, who is a personal trainer, fell for one of her clients when the girls were in elementary school, and this led to a divorce. After this, Jacob had relationships with a series of women, often several at one time, and began to identify as polyamorous when a friend from his men's group introduced him to my work. When Jacob's older daughter was a senior in high school, he remarried, again choosing an open marriage. Jacob's older daughter, Rachael, like Nora and Jim's daughter, Carla, is a very monogamous lesbian who graduated from college with high honors. His younger daughter, Georgia, is currently applying to graduate schools in psychology and, for the first time since she started dating at fifteen, has managed to take a breather from coupling up and is without a steady boyfriend. "I've tried to stay single before," she disclosed, "but it's not easy. The guys kind of pressure you to be exclusive, and when you get really close, it's just easier."

Jacob says that he never discussed the women in his life with his children until the last couple of years but that he didn't hide anything either. He says that Georgia had an issue with all those women taking away some of her precious time with Dad, but otherwise she hadn't seen it as a problem. The main complaint from Georgia was this: "It was weird, Dad, because you always had these different smells on you, and some of them I really didn't like!"

I was starting to get the picture that polyamory can be challenging for teens and young adults even when they've been raised in polyamorous families and even when they're not opposed to it. If polyamory was challenging for Raymond, I was pretty sure it would be challenging for any young adult. I decided to ask my own twenty-one-year-old daughter who was born into an open relationship and is now studying psychology at Stanford University what she thought. Once again, I was amazed by how mature and articulate this generation of young adults can be. I certainly don't remember being mature enough at twenty-one to know I was immature, and if I had known, I'm sure I wouldn't have admitted it to my mother or any other adult.

Alana wasn't sure when she first became aware of polyamory. Her father and I were appearing on national television talking about our open marriage by the time she was three, but she was apparently oblivious to our open relationship if not to our absence. We were grateful that my mother was living with us, so we could easily leave her at home with Grandma while we flew to New York, say our sound bites, and fly home. It was a pretty big deal to us because we always got shredded by the host, who would sometimes apologize afterward and say it was a job requirement. But to a three-year-old, the details were irrelevant. It was simply a matter of "I didn't like it when you went out without me. Otherwise, I didn't think anything about it. I didn't pay much attention. I thought your friends were weird because they ate raw and vegan food and meditated and belly danced, stuff like that. I really didn't see and wasn't interested in their sex lives. I felt different when you got divorced because my best friends' parents weren't divorced, but that's all."

So what does she think about polyamory now? "I think polyamory is fine, there's nothing wrong with it, but it's not a good idea for most people because the way our society teaches people to view relationships is not compatible with polyamory, and when they try it, they get jealous. Most people I know think polyamory would never work for them because they'd get jealous. Friends with benefits is popular, but that's viewed differently, it's just hooking up in a pretty shallow way. It's accepted by people, but when they get involved, they want commitment."

Alana reminds me that when she went away to college, she tried to have an open relationship with the boyfriend she'd had the last two years of high school, but it didn't work. When I asked her why, she replied, "Because we were eighteen, immature, insecure, and had poor communication skills. We should have just broken up and been friends, but we were too codependent to separate. He's a particularly jealous person, and it just didn't work." What about the next boyfriend, who left for law school last fall? I asked. "Oh, we talked about it, but he's a serial monogamist. He said,

'That's just how I do it.' End of conversation." And the current boyfriend, whom she met just before leaving the country for a study abroad program? "He's definitely more open. His aunt and uncle run a summer camp for nonmonogamous people, and his parents met at a hippie commune in the seventies. But his dad couldn't deal with jealousy, so they moved to the suburbs and had a normal family life. He now lives at a Buddhist retreat center and has other girlfriends which I'm not really thrilled about, but I'm out of the country, and we agreed not to be exclusive, so I can't really complain."

Alana goes on to tell me that many of the students in her study-abroad program are in a similar situation and miserable. "Either they've broken up because they knew they were going to be apart but they're not really over each other, or they're trying to be open since they're so far away, but they're jealous."

What's interesting to me is that most of the young adults I know who were raised in child-centered polyamorous families seem to end up giving a higher priority to bonding and sustained intimacy than to freedom, whether they are male or female. While they often attempt both, they seem willing to go for serial monogamy because its continued cultural dominance provides greater ease in intimate connections with partners raised to believe in monogamy. Those who are more determined to pursue radical multipartner lifestyles whatever the cost or who are hungry for sexual variety to make up for a sexually repressed adolescence seem to have a greater need to rebel against the culture norms than the children of the last generation of polyamorous pioneers. This pattern also seems to hold true for the children of more mainstream families who are open with their children about their polyamorous relationships.

SETTING A CONTEXT FOR CHILDREN

Kelly is a corporate executive with a multinational company based in Vancouver, Canada. He's a youthful forty-seven-year-old who has been happily married to Eileen, his high school sweetheart for twenty-five years. They have an eleven-year-old daughter and two sons who are eighteen and nineteen. This family looks like the most traditional, child-centered family anyone could imagine. Eileen is a stay-at-home mom who has spent years chauffeuring the children to various activities, helping them with their homework, and preparing special holiday treats. Despite the demands of his work, Kelly puts a high priority on family life, and when he's not traveling between corporate offices, he always joins in family dinners, where the art of meaningful conversation is carefully taught. Like Nora and Jim, Kelly and Eileen were virgins when they got together and wanted to expand their sexual experience without breaking up their marriage. Nine years ago, when Kelly and Eileen decided to open their marriage, they realized they needed to prepare the children for a new way of life.

Kelly recalls that "the whole issue about kids was a big one for us. The kids were two, nine, and ten at the time and never exposed to anything other than normal family life. We were very proactive in preparing a context for them to be comfortable with what we were doing so they wouldn't have any surprises. We were aware that the picture of extramarital relationships they would get from films or TV was a negative one, all about secret affairs, drama, and unhappiness. It's always a bad thing, it's ugly, that's the dominant picture kids get. So while we never sat the kids down and directly talked about what we were doing, we made sure they knew there were no secrets going on between Mom and Dad and no hiding.

"As our relationships with others evolved, we never hid our warmth for other people in our lives. We talked to the children about how much we were looking forward to seeing certain people and how much we loved them. So they were not surprised to see us hugging or being affectionate with each other in the kitchen while waiting for the water to boil for the potatoes. We had no problem expressing warmth and love in front of the kids. Of course we didn't feel each other up; we didn't do that as a couple either. We didn't talk about our sex lives and who was sleeping where, but we didn't hide it either. We talked openly about our lovers to the kids. We told them how much we enjoy spending time together or that so and so had called. We went to a lot of effort to set a context so that the kids never needed to feel uncomfortable about what was evolving in our relationships with others. We found that the kids tended to be warm and accepting with whomever we were warm and accepting with ourselves. There were times when we felt self-conscious, but mostly we just normalized the whole thing."

About two years after opening their marriage, they met Erica. After dating for three years, Erica moved into the family home. "Erica was more like a favorite aunt than a parent," Kelly explains. "She was just remarkable with the children, and they adore her. Even now, sometimes she stays with them when we go away." The threesome ended after six months of living together, and each of the three has a slightly different take on why it ended, but they're still close friends who talk every week and occasionally visit with Erica and her new partner.

Kelly emphasizes, "We felt it was very important never to lie to the kids, not even a white lie, so if they asked, where did we meet this person, we'd say, on the Internet, which was the truth, not at work or some other cover-up. We rarely get questions from the kids because we give them all the information they need. But if they ask, we answer truthfully. If I spent the weekend away with Erica and they asked, where did she sleep, I'd say, she slept with me."

Kelly has known Selena for about eight years, and they've been lovers for five, but she's only recently met the kids when she came to visit the family for a week. Eileen is slowly warming up to Selena, Kelly says, but prefers to stay with just friendship for now. Kelly explains that his relationship with Selena began while the family was living in England, and he would see Selena when he was in Vancouver on business. Selena has three children of her own who spend most weekends with their father, and they're not at all ready to tackle the complexities of bringing the two families together, although I get the feeling that Kelly would like to if he could figure out the right context.

I asked Kelly if he'd discussed polyamory with his oldest son Trent, who is now nineteen and has a girlfriend. Kelly replied that Trent is aware that some of their friends are also lovers, but it just hasn't come up with the younger ones. "Mike has never been very communicative, he's more of a geek, and while Sally is nosier than the boys were, she's really more concerned with her own life so far." Kelly continued, "I've always had a close relationship with Trent, and he's brought me questions about sex since he was eight or nine. When he was younger we would shower together, and that's when we would talk. So if he wanted to talk to me, he'd say, 'Dad, can we take a shower?' He'd ask me about things he'd heard on the playground that he wanted to know more about. Once some kids called him a fag, so he wanted to know what that meant, and then he wanted to know how gay men had sex."

For the past two years, Trent has had a long-distance relationship with a girl who's away at boarding school. Kelly describes Trent as "a very good looking, outgoing, talented kid who plays in a band, and he always has a string of girls following him around. When we saw him starting to spend time with another girl, we did have a talk with him about whether he was about to create some drama with the two girls and advised him to communicate openly with both of them. We told him he'd have to decide how to handle it, but he should be honorable and not lie or withhold information and practice safe sex. We did mention polyamory, or sexual friendship, as possibilities and pointed out the advantages and responsibilities that go with different choices. I'm not sure exactly what he decided, but he slept over at the other girl's house, and that was followed by a series of lengthy phone calls with the girlfriend who's away at school. We were concerned that all the time processing was cutting into his time for homework and were relieved when they broke up."

I loved the practical, down-to-earth way that Kelly and Eileen managed what could have been a rocky transition for their children from a traditional monogamous marriage to a polyamorous lifestyle. It was an added bonus that their life experience then allowed them to support their teenage son in making ethical and responsible choices for himself. For families with small children, the polyamorous context is often set from birth, so it doesn't seem alien to the children unless it clashes with the larger culture. Living in a socially liberal area is one way to avoid this clash, but crossing national boundaries is another way to circumvent rigid cultural norms, as illustrated in the following histories.

BRINGING UP BABY

Juliette, Roland, Laurel, and their one-year-old daughter, Maya, make polyamory look about as normal—and easy—as anyone could imagine. But then none of them are teenagers. All three adults are in their early forties and are self-employed freelancers. Juliette and Roland met and fell in love while both were working in Washington, D.C., in the mid-1990s. At the time, Juliette was married to another man, and it was Roland who first suggested they try a polyamorous relationship, but Juliette's husband didn't like the idea. Eventually, they divorced, and she and Roland were married. Juliette says that the first ten years of their marriage were spent learning how to have an open relationship, moving to Spain, and trying to conceive—without success.

Two and a half years ago, they met Laurel, who had recently moved to Spain from France, through the polyamory network Juliette had started.

Roland and Laurel were six months into their love affair when Laurel accidentally got pregnant. Roland was apprehensive about Juliette's reaction to the news, but, as it turned out, she was just as delighted as the other two, perhaps because after some experience with medical interventions for infertility, she recognized this as an opportunity to bring a baby into their lives in a less expensive and more enjoyable way. They quickly decided that they all wanted to raise this baby and moved in together a few months before Maya was born. Juliette says they all get along very harmoniously and take an equal share in the parenting responsibilities. In a recent newspaper interview, Laurel attributed their success to good communication.

I spoke with Juliette and Roland via Skype at their Barcelona home recently, and they told me that "it's amazing how not different it is raising a baby in a triad." Of course, they've never raised a baby any other way so probably wouldn't believe me if I told them how much easier it can be to have an "extra" adult in the house, but they did say they're happy to find it's getting less demanding now that Maya is beyond infancy. Roland says the hardest part was having virtually no time for himself while juggling a job, a baby, and two women. This triad believes in being open to the flow and is currently considering adding Laurel's new boyfriend, who lives in Amsterdam, to the family. Their only agreement, apart from honesty with each other, is that they'll wait six months to a year, until the new relationship energy has worn off with a new lover before making any big decisions about the future. Roland emphasizes that he is heterosexual, so, while he prefers to have friendship and mutual respect with his partners' lovers, he's not looking for sexual intimacy with a man. Rather, they "must respect and treat my partners well. I've had to hold my tongue at times with men I didn't like being around and didn't think were treating Juliette well, but eventually it didn't work out with them anyway. I try to allow the women to discover this themselves, and I hope to do the same with my daughter when she grows up. People need to be allowed to find things out for themselves and not be told what to do."

Roland is as surprised as anyone to find himself "married" to two women. He always assumed he'd be sharing Juliette with another man instead of vice versa. "I've only been with three women in my life," he says, "and I'm still with two of them, whereas Juliette has had a number of boyfriends." Roland says he always believed women can have multiple loves, but he really wasn't that interested in finding another woman for himself. It just happened.

When I asked Roland how he escaped the usual male programming, he immediately pointed to his cross-cultural background. "Moving from country to country as a child, I never felt the kind of peer pressure that what society and friends are telling you is what you have to do," he explains. "I had few friends and was always an outsider socially." Roland also feels that his birth order, being the middle child of three, meant that from the very beginning of his life, he was accustomed to sharing the love of his parents with siblings, so he's comfortable with not being the center of attention and knows there's always enough love to go around. Roland also mentioned the Christian values he was raised with, especially Christ's emphasis on unconditional love, as an important influence.

As foreigners in Spain—both Juliette and Laurel are Americans, and Roland is British but lived in Africa, Colombia, and Mexico before his family moved to the United States when he was a teen—they feel graced with a freedom from social norms that the Spaniards might hesitate to extend to their own kin. They're close friends with another polyamorous family who live nearby but are originally from Germany. In terms of the reactions of their own families, Juliette tells me that Roland's family has been the most supportive, and this was a big surprise to them because his parents are quite religious. As mainstream Methodists, they've apparently taken to heart the teachings of Jesus. Both Juliette's and Laurel's parents are divorced and not very happy about the situation, but their mothers seem to be getting over their original upset.

Roland and Juliette bristle a bit when I ask if they've thought about what they would do about custody in the event of a breakup. "Couples don't usually think about future breakups when they have children, and we don't either," they retort. "I have less fear in my heart about this than the standard monogamous couple. I'm not really worried about it," Roland continues, clearly finding it tedious that everyone asks this question, but he relents and says, "We'd move, to another country if necessary, to be close enough to continue having a relationship with Maya."

Kamala and Michael, whom we first met in chapter 2, live in suburban San Diego with their son, Devon, and with Michael's dad. Ever since Devon was born three years ago, Kamala has been hosting poly potlucks and other workshops and social events at their home. I first met Kamala about ten years ago when she was a popular "hot bi babe" in the growing San Diego poly community. Kamala is a slender, high-energy woman who seems to juggle her family, numerous lovers, and a booming business with ease. When I asked her to tell me what life is like for her as a polyamorous mom, she readily agreed. Kamala enthusiastically described how thrilled Devon is to welcome both old and new friends and lovers, whom she introduces to him as "auntie" or "uncle," into their home. He often becomes the "doorman" at events like the monthly poly potluck, running to answer the doorbell for arriving guests, all of whom know him and greet him warmly.

Devon is usually the only child in this sea of loving adults, but he doesn't seem to mind. He happily takes his place in the introduction circle where people say their names and are asked to name a flower that expresses how they're feeling. It's rare for other children to attend these events, although Kamala says she doesn't discourage it. Kamala proudly relates how Devon, who is barely three, understands the game and shouts "Daisy!" when it's his turn. After dinner when the group discussion gets deeper, Devon goes off to spend time with Grandpa, who is the "nighttime nanny" after the full-time nanny goes home for the evening. "The reason we don't include Devon is not because of the content," Kamala says, "but because of his attention span." Kamala reports that Michael's dad is very liberal and has no gripe with their lifestyle, although he has suggested that as Devon gets older, they should put an addition onto their suburban San Diego house to allow him more space from the hubbub.

At three, Devon is too young for much in the way of verbal explanation of a poly lifestyle, but he loves to watch the recorded television spots of Mom and Dad discussing polyamory because he's in some of them. Kamala recalls that he has asked questions when he happens on Mom or Dad engaged with another partner but usually takes it in stride. For example, when he's entered their bedroom while she's with another lover, he might ask, "Where's Dad?" And Kamala will matter-of-factly respond, "He's in the other room with Auntie June." Between them, Kamala and Michael have about ten other lovers, and Kamala is gratified to find that "their love for me spills over to my son."

While their lifestyle no doubt sounds outrageous to many people, Kamala is very public about her life and often appears on television talk shows along with various intimate friends. She says she's unconcerned about the possibility of government interference because there's no one in their families or social circle who would make a complaint and Devon is so obviously a happy and healthy child. She says they own their home, pay their taxes, and just don't anticipate any problems. However, Kamala reports that many of the critical comments on her blog do concern children. After her appearance on the *Tyra Banks Show*, a woman wrote that "with all these sex addicts coming in and out of your house, how long do you think it will be before someone molests your child?" Kamala was genuinely shocked by this comment, telling me, "I'd be much more concerned in a community where people are not bringing so much light and healing to their sexuality as we do here."

CUSTODY ISSUES

Although it's quite rare, there have been some well-publicized cases in the United States in which poly families or communities have had their children taken away either temporarily or permanently, but even a temporary issue can have long-term repercussions. When I asked Roland and Juliette, the expatriates living in Spain, whether they had any concerns about losing custody of their child after being so public about their triadic parenting, they were shocked. Roland explained, "Because of the recency of the Franco regime, there's still a sense of quiet rebellion about the government interfering in people's private lives, and the government knows this too. It's inconceivable that the government would come in and take a child just because the parents were polyamorous."

But in 1998 in Memphis, Tennessee, that's exactly what happened. April, Shane, and Chris were a happy triad, all in their twenties, who were raising April's preschooler from a previous relationship. April and Shane were legally married and living with April's additional male partner Chris when the threesome agreed to appear on MTV's *Sex in the '90s* series. The child's Christian grandmother was outraged by their polyamorous (and pagan) lifestyle, and a judge ordered that the child be removed from her stay-at-home mother's home and put in custody of the grandmother. The legal battle went on for two years, with Chris moving out in an effort to convince authorities to allow the child to return to her mother. Despite the testimony of four different court-appointed experts who concluded that the girl belonged with her mother and an appeal by April's attorney on constitutional grounds, the Tennesse judge refused to rule in her favor. April eventually declared herself "unfit" due to poverty and let the grandmother keep the child.

In a more recent custody case, another Tennessee mother was at risk of losing custody of her ten-year-old child, but with the help of the Sexual

Freedom League Defense Fund, she got her daughter back without having to leave her triad. The Defense Fund's website[9] has some useful advice for people contemplating polyamorous parenthood, which includes such considerations as deciding who will be listed as parents on the birth certificate, voluntary guardianship (which adds legal guardians without displacing biological parents), estate planning, medical insurance, and custody, property, and visitation agreements in the event of "divorce."

The Washington, D.C.–based polyamorous community known as the Finders lost custody of their children in 1987 but only temporarily in this extraordinarily bizarre case. However, the sensational newspaper coverage, filled with lurid but contrived accusations that they were a satanic cult, along with rumors of involvement by the Central Intelligence Agency (CIA), soon led to the demise of the entire community, which had been active for several decades. My friend Michael, who is now in his forties, joined the community right out of high school in the late 1970s and was at the center of the controversy.

As a young man, Michael was attracted to the group by its charismatic leader who became a father figure for him and also by the group's philosophy, which he perceived as doing everything the reverse of the way it was done in the mainstream because clearly the "normal" way of doing things didn't work very well. Michael's parents had tried having an open marriage as part of their human potential explorations in the 1970s but, like many couples in that era, ended up getting divorced. Both parents were too absorbed by their own dilemmas to pay much attention to their children. Michael describes his father as a pot-smoking womanizer and his mother as withdrawn and less available than Michael would have liked. As a self-described nerdy teenager, handsome but too shy and intellectual to be popular with girls, Michael had a difficult adolescence. He was disillusioned both with the mainstream society and by what he'd seen of the "ESThole's" way of managing relationships.

As Michael describes it, "The idea behind the Finders was to share everything—money, clothes, food, and also sex partners. It wasn't polyamory as I think of it now because we were not necessarily drawn to each other; we were drawn to the leader who would orchestrate different games."

The number of adults in the group ranged from about ten to twenty during Michael's years there. All were white and mostly well-educated professionals between twenty and forty-something years old. There were a total of seven children, all except one of whom were born in the community.

Michael recalls that "one day the leader would tell all the women to pick a man, get married, and have children. Another day he might tell everyone to get divorced." Sometimes he would wake them up in the middle of the night and send them on a "mission," so they learned to always keep a suitcase packed with essentials. Michael remembers that "everything was always changing, and it was fun for the adults, but in retrospect I think it was confusing for the children. It was one of these spontaneous, midnight directives which instructed all the women to fly to California and the men to drive there in two vans with the six children. We were all to rendezvous in California, but along the way we stopped in Florida."

One day, Michael and another man were in a public playground with six scruffy-looking children, only one of whom was his biological child, when they attracted the attention of the police, who suspected a kidnapping or worse. Six children with two women probably would not have been a remarkable sight, but the police took the two men into custody and placed the children in foster care. After forty days in the county jail, all charges were dropped and the men released, but meanwhile the case had made national headlines, and the children were fairly traumatized.

In a rare 1998 interview,[10] founder Marion Petty, who died not long after giving the interview, said that he began to keep "open house" in the 1930s and over the years hosted many well-known counterculture figures as well as a handful of followers who were with him for over twenty-five years. He acknowledged that he did have CIA contacts during World War II and that his wife later worked as an administrator for the CIA but denied that his CIA connections explain why the case against Michael was dropped and the children returned to their parents.

The whole truth may never be known, but Michael, who I've known well for over a decade, says that the case was fabricated in typical tabloid fashion even though it was reported by respectable daily papers. For example, pictures of white-clothed "satanic rituals" were from a Halloween party, nudity was just part of their lifestyle and had nothing to do with pedophilia, and sacrificial animals were part of an educational project to teach the children about raising animals for food. The whole case is one of the strangest ever to make the news and has given conspiracy buffs on both sides of the fence plenty of ammunition, but I tend to believe Michael when he says that while the Finders was surely a cult—and a polyamorous one at that—there was no child abuse or buying and selling of children involved. As for the CIA, who knows?

Most of the members left the community in the aftermath of the scandal. One former member who had no children of his own but became a kind of surrogate father to them all still keeps an "open house" in the San Francisco Bay Area, and the grown children often visit him. Now young adults, they seem to have emerged no more scathed than your average twenty-something-year-old. Michael's own son, now twenty-four, graduated from college with a major in theater and currently works as a substitute teacher in an inner-city school system. Michael says that one boy who had the most challenging time in a series of foster homes ended up joining the military and is now serving in Iraq. To Michael, this is a failure, but for many Americans, it's something to be proud of.

While the simple fact of polyamory can be alarming to those raised to believe in monogamy, polyamorous communities with children can easily be seen as an even bigger threat to society. Even though few have been as controversial as the Finders, these communities sometimes have challenges interfacing with the outside world, but still the children seem to do at least as well as those in the average nuclear family.

CHILDREN IN POLYAMOROUS COMMUNITIES

The ZEGG community relocated from the Black Forest to Belzig, Germany, in 1990 when the Berlin Wall came down and a former Stasi camp in what had been East Germany became available at a very reasonable price. We'll discuss this community in more detail in chapter 9, but for now let's just say that it was founded on the premise that "a free society needs free love," which is one of their popular slogans. Currently, there are about fifteen children living at ZEGG, while an earlier generation of young people who were raised there are now in their twenties and off on their journeys into adulthood. Ina, who has been part of ZEGG from the beginning, told me that this first group of children lived together in the Children's House when they were in their teens, much like the children of the Osho ashram. There were four or five of them, she recalls, and they were very physically affectionate together, snuggling and touching a lot but not having sex with each other. In fact, Ina tells me that they all chose not to become fully sexual at all until their late teens. The group is still quite close, like brothers and sisters, and stay in touch via Facebook and instant messaging. Some are now at the university or working in Berlin, which is only an hour away, so they often come to visit. Others have gone to live at ZEGG's sister community of Tamera in Portugal and have children of their own

The children now at ZEGG don't live separately from the adults but meet daily at the children's house after school and sometimes on Saturdays and usually have lunch there as well. The house and adult staff are provided by the community who feel it's important that the children be supported to build their own community. The parents at ZEGG also have a close community with each other and support each other in being parents.

Most of the children live with either both parents or their mothers, but it varies according to the needs of each family. One boy decided that he wanted to live in a larger living group where his friends lived instead of in a small house with his mother, and she supported that, though she still visits with him every day. Sometimes a daughter will live with her mother and a son with his father if the parents are no longer together as a couple, which is often the case. Usually, the parents remain good friends even after a separation and may go on holidays together as a family or to visit grandparents, so the children are still held in a secure family after a divorce. Still, Ina feels that it's challenging to create enough stability in open relationships to make a safe container for kids.

Over the years, she's observed that if the parents feel good in their open relationship, it's easy for the children to accept new partners. If one parent feels neglected or unhappy about it, then the children don't like it. Another difficulty is that some of the parents in the local neighborhood won't allow their children to play at the homes of the ZEGG children; they think it's too dangerous because of scandalous reports in the press in earlier years. But on the whole, ZEGG and its children are accepted. Ina explains that "we've been here eighteen years, so they see that in spite of what they may have read or heard about us, we take care of our gardens and our buildings. We're not as strange as they may have thought at first."

Ina, who has no children of her own, says that before living at ZEGG, she thought it was normal for teens to be in conflict with their parents because that's how she grew up. Now she realizes that it's possible for teens to have deep friendship and open communication with their parents. Often the teens will choose another adult in the community who is not their parent to bring questions about sex and relationships. All the adult women participate in circles to encourage the young women to value their womanhood and answer their questions about love and sex. Part of the gift of living in community is the opportunity to play an important role in children's lives without the demands and responsibility of being a full-time parent. Ina says that this has very much been the case at ZEGG, where there are relatively few children partly because in the early years at ZEGG, there was the idea that you had to be almost perfect, an ideal woman, to be a mother.

ZEGG founder Dieter Duhm may have gotten the idea for the children's house from the Osho ashram in Pune, India, which he visited in the 1970s. Jivana Kennedy is an American woman who spent several years at the ashram. Her own children never lived there, as their father took custody of them before she went to the ashram in her late thirties, but she reports that "from everything I've heard, those kids grew into the sanest and most creative teenagers anyone would want to be around—sensual and free but not crazed from the distortions that arise from lack of information and repression."

While Osho often praised conscious monogamy as a very evolved form of relationship, he was a severe critic of the traditional family, saying that it was "no longer relevant for the new humanity that is just being born." While acknowledging that families have helped people survive, he said that it was rare for a family to be loving, joyous, and free. Most were a "necessary evil," which "corrupts the human mind" and breeds neuroses. Instead, he proposed that children belong to the commune as a whole, where they would "have more opportunities to grow with many more kinds of people" while their biological parents were freed to love each other or not without clinging together for the sake of the children.[11] In the early days of the ashram, Osho's theories were put into practice.

Jivana recalls that in the ashram, the children generally lived together with the most loving adults being the caretakers of the kids. "All the kids knew exactly who their parents were and had special time with them, but the rest of the time the parents were freed to play their social role, whatever that was, and the kids were socialized together with loving and nurturing supervision. Stories would float around about how five- and six-year-olds would touch and fondle each other and sometimes even attempt penetration, but no one made any fuss about it. It was considered natural. The adults were in their own process of awakening to the unnaturalness of the uptight conditions in which they had been raised and were committed to *not* laying those trips on the kids."

"Osho would often talk about teenage sex and how it was the most innocent, the most raw and pure of sexual experiences, and how it could help to blossom people into sexually loving adults when it was not thwarted and laden with fear and moral judgment or hidden in secrecy and shame. When it made sense to have conversations about birth control and STDs [sexually transmitted diseases], those talks were all handled intelligently and with love and met with little resistance from the kids," Jivana concludes.

I know of one European teen who refused to live at the Ashram because she chafed at the rules and restrictions, which were not sexual in nature but applied to dress, schedules, spiritual practices, and the like and which she found oppressive. Instead, she stayed in the town and met with her beloved sanyasin father at the ashram gate. In chapter 5, we heard the story of Rainah, who feels that her teen years at the Osho ashram made her who she is today.

The Kerista commune, based in San Francisco and discussed at length in chapter 3, is another polyamorous group where the child-to-adult ratio was very low, as at ZEGG and the Osho ashram. After seeing how much time, money, and energy were needed to parent the two very carefully planned children born into Kerista, the commune decided that two children for thirty adults was enough and required all Keristan men to undergo vasectomies. I'd long since lost track of the two girls born into the Kerista commune who were in their early teens when the commune broke up, although they continued to live in a smaller group marriage for a time. The last time I'd seen them was shortly after the commune broke up, and they would sometimes babysit for me when my own daughter was small. After so many years living in a fishbowl, many former Keristans now want privacy, so I wasn't able to interview either of these young women, who are now in their twenties. I did get a report from a personal friend who told me that one is just about to graduate from medical school, and the other is monogamously married with children of her own and living a normal life in rural Hawaii. Any parent anywhere in the world would have plenty to brag about having children like these.

One of the few thoroughly polyamorous intentional communities in the United States had a strong focus on children. I say "had" because while the remaining three members are still child focused, they are no longer polyamorous. In the end, their desire to expand their service to children beyond their own family led them to abandon the practice of nonmonogamy. They're still convinced that multiple parenting in a communal environment is good for children but say that they eventually found the interface with the larger society too difficult and limiting.

Heavily influenced by the Asian cultures visited by their male founder during his many years of travel, this group, which now prefers to remain anonymous, came together in the mid-1990s and were together as a community for the next ten years. During this time, there were anywhere from six to twelve adults and five to eight children, some of them born at home in the community. Three of the adults, two men and a woman whom I'll call Mara, still live together, along with her three children, ages four, ten, and thirteen, each by different fathers. The oldest, now twenty-one, recently moved out of the family home after attending the local community college. He's currently off traveling the world and was unavailable for an interview. Mara, his stepmother, describes him as very responsible but definitely choosing an alternative lifestyle.

I spent several days with this group in their early days in the late 1990s. My partner and I were traveling in their area, and a mutual friend suggested that we visit them. The visit, which was originally planned for a few hours, kept extending itself, as I found their whole approach to parenting and relationships fascinating. When they invited us to spend the night, we readily agreed. At that time, they were gradually carving out a homestead in the jungle. It was by far the most rustic living (as opposed to camping) environment I'd been in up to that point. They had a large outdoor kitchen that was the daytime hub for the community and one large structure that they called the "birthing hut" with a roof, screened walls, and a dirt floor covered with large rugs where everyone slept. The only fully enclosed structure was a small air-conditioned room that housed their computers and office equipment. I still remember the sense of "coming home" that I felt sleeping on futons in the birthing hut amidst the whole tribe of children and adults while listening to the sounds of the jungle outside.

One of the community members explained that the birthing hut was originally built so that they would have a clean, dry place where the women could give birth, but everyone liked the space so much that it eventually became the nighttime hub for the community. At the time I visited, all the children were small and would sleep with their parents in "family beds." Those few adults who were not biological parents generally slept in another area of the birthing hut, and in the center was a large open area for making music and art and conversing with each other. Mara told me that if people wanted to have sex, they went out in pairs to little huts some distance away, but mostly people gathered in the big room every evening, and she felt that this was the greatest benefit to the children. During the day, the children would go around together in "little packs" learning and playing with supervision from only a few adults, but at night everyone was together.

"The kids gained so much; they developed magnificent talents! When you live with artists, you become one. The kids learned to cut, sew, paint, draw, and talk at very early ages. People said they had extraordinarily advanced communication skills, and they could converse easily with adults." Mara concedes that the same is true to some extent of neighboring monogamous families who also practice the "continuum concept," but advanced communication skills is one trait that keeps popping up as I talk to polyamorous parents about their children.

One of the things that intrigued me about this community was that the women tried to conceive around the same time so that they could breast-feed each other's babies. I'd been a breast-feeding mom myself not so many years before, so I immediately understood the practicality of this custom, which made caring for another mother's infant or toddler in her absence much easier and more natural. But there was more to it than convenience. Part of their philosophy was that our cultural obsession with monogamy begins at our mother's breasts. Either literally or figuratively, we learn that one person—usually Mommy—is the source of love, nourishment, nurturing, and safety—all those things we later seek in a romantic partner. They theorized that if they instead conditioned their children to receive love—and mother's milk—from more than one nurturing caretaker, they would be conditioning their children to bond with more than one beloved or "multisource" later in life. It's too early to know whether these children will grow up to be jealousy-free polyamorous adults, and, in any case, it's certainly not a controlled experiment, but I found it an interesting concept.

According to Mara, the remaining members of the group eventually decided to "single source," as they call monogamy, because "polyamory was too much of a button pusher for people, and we're not into a cover-up." They now have a very public lifestyle as an educational co-op for young children and were a charter school site for three years. Mara is currently an elementary school teacher and feels vulnerable to public scrutiny. As she puts it, "The cocoon in which we had our poly family was too confining after a while. We wanted a larger context for our work with children. The social confines of the poly family were tight, and we didn't want to risk either losing custody of the children or having the children encounter problems in dealing with the outside world. But when the community broke up, it was like having a phantom limb. The others were supposed to be there, but they weren't."

Mara feels that the community struggled because they attracted too many wounded people with histories of sexual and physical abuse. "There was not a strong enough 'center' to hold a container for all the healing they needed to do," she says, but critics feel that the community was too extreme and required too much of people. As in many monogamous breakups, there is often more than one side to the story or even more than one story for each person at different points in time. Whatever worked or didn't work will probably never be known, but I have to admire these folks for putting it all on the line in their determination to find a better way to raise their children.

CHILD-CENTERED FAMILY

My impression, after examining what little evidence we have, is that it is not polyamory per se but rather the extent to which the family and the culture it's embedded in are child centered (or not) that influences the health and well-being of the children. The 2008 CBS television series *Swingtown* provides an excellent example of how this distinction impacts children. While the story line is fictional, the program was created by a man whose own parents had an open marriage, and the characters are amazingly true to life if somewhat stereotypical portraits of "two generations of friends and neighbors as they forge intimate connections and explore new freedoms during the culturally transformative decade of the 1970's," according to the CBS promotional information.

Swingtown follows three sets of couples: one of them fun-loving seasoned swingers with no children; one upwardly mobile and open-minded pair who are conscientious parents with two healthy, normal teenage children; and one moralistic and judgemental pair who have a sexually repressed teenage son. There is also a neighboring single mom whose teenage daughter is left to fend for herself while the mother indulges in drugs, alcohol, and sexual adventures.

The couple who exhibit the most turbulence are the two who make themselves vulnerable to the turmoil of questioning their values and experimenting with opening their marriage. However, they never allow their inner turmoil or adults-only recreation to interfere with their ability to parent effectively. They consistently provide parental support and supervision while allowing an appropriate level of freedom and autonomy to their son and daughter. Their son ends up taking on a protective role with the girl next door, who runs away from home only to find that her self-absorbed mother hasn't noticed. His older sister explores her own sexuality and intellectual interests and refuses to cave in to her cute but not-so-bright boyfriend's possessiveness. Meanwhile, the "normal" couple, though good intentioned, are exposed as smothering, controlling, and overprotective parents whose son is developing into a misogynist, pornography-addicted loser.

While the Moral Majority often complains that the media have a liberal bias, in my view *Swingtown* is just telling it like it is. I doubt that such an honest and accurate portrayal of nonmonogamy could have been shown on network television prior to the twenty-first century.

8

COMING-OUT ISSUES

The term *coming out* has been popularized by its use in the gay, lesbian, and bisexual communities to describe the process of telling the truth about oneself and one's sexual orientation. Someone who has not yet come out is said to be *in the closet*. These concepts apply quite well to people with a polyamorous relationship orientation. However, as we shall see, there are significant differences as well as significant parallels with the homosexual and bisexual experiences. Some polyamorous people find that the challenges of coming out are even more threatening than dealing with jealousy, while others simply skirt the whole matter by not taking on a polyamorous identity even though they are engaged with multiple partners in an ongoing and consensual way.

COMING OUT IS A PROCESS

Coming out is an ongoing process that occurs gradually over many years. It includes first recognizing that you do not conform to the relevant norm—in this case, admitting that you are willing and able to love more than one person at a time. Once you've recognized yourself as not necessarily being monogamous and not wanting to lie about it, you then have to sort out what you *do* want and learn to accept and love yourself as you are. Part of

coming out to yourself involves finding a label, name, or identity that more
accurately describes who you are or at least finding a way to see yourself
and think about your desires and behaviors that corresponds to the reality
of how you show up in the world.

People who've never thought about it might think that admitting to being polyamorous or accepting oneself as polyamorous would be a simple
matter, but most us of have been thoroughly indoctrinated to believe that
we should be monogamous. Although this is rapidly changing, polyamory
is still considered deviant. Many people have also developed judgments
based on experiences with other people's unethical or disharmonious nonmonogamous styles of relating and are reluctant to associate themselves
with these negative examples. Consequently, people are often more likely
to expend energy trying to squeeze themselves into a monogamous mold
than considering the possibility that it's really okay to relate to more than
one person at a time.

I recently granted an interview for a podcast. The interviewer clearly
had a negative attitude about polyamory, so I asked her what she thought
of when she thought of polyamory. She immediately said, "Thank you for
asking me that!" and began telling me that when she asked people what
they were looking for in relationships, men usually said that they wanted
freedom to date lots of women, whereas women often said they were looking for "the one." In her own life, she'd struggled with a partner who'd
wanted to be polyamorous but whom she didn't feel she could trust to be
honest with her about what he was doing. In addition, she was horrified
by the sometimes insensitive and manipulative ways in which she saw men
trying to impose their polyamorous agendas on the women in their lives.
She saw polyamory as a weapon in the war between the sexes that was most
often employed by men who were "unwilling to commit." There was no
way she wanted to identify herself as polyamorous.

Nevertheless, it turned out that she now found herself choosing to be
involved with an openly polyamorous man. "I met him at a party, and he
told me that he had a girlfriend and that he wanted to be intimate with me
and asked me to call him," she explained. "So I did call him, and I met the
girlfriend, and she was fine with my seeing him, so we got together. We
have a great time—he's fun, he's mature, he's sexy. But now he's splitting
up with the girlfriend, and I don't know how that will turn out. I kind of
liked being the other woman. I guess I'll have to take another look at polyamory." This woman was more willing than most to let go of a belief that

was no longer congruent with her experience, but still she was struggling with her identity.

Once you're clear about who you are, the next important step in coming out is beginning to let other people know you are polyamorous. Whether you choose to label yourself polyamorous is less important than choosing to let others know you are not committed to monogamy, at least on a "need-to-know" basis. Often the first people who are told are people whom you know will support, accept, or at least not care very much about your sexual or relationship orientation. Usually, the last people you're ready to come out to are the people who count the most—lovers, employers, parents, and family.

For Kelly, deciding who to come out to is not so much a matter of how close he is to people but rather how open minded they are. As he puts it, "I don't mind doing something out of the ordinary, but I prepare the context for people before telling them because you have to equip people to be able to hear you, or it's not worth sharing. If we know they're just going to be hurt or shocked and we're not prepared to invest the time and energy to give them a tool kit to understand, it's better not to tell. The criteria is whether they'll accept the tool kit instead of seeing us through their lens of fear or judgment."

Other people find it easier to just stop keeping any secrets from anyone. Otherwise, new situations continually arise where you will be faced with decisions about how to present yourself, but once all the important people in your life have been told, the fear of discovery diminishes.

Polyamorous people are perhaps the last sexual "minority" to come out of hiding. In an age when homosexuals demand church weddings and some cities have passed domestic partner ordinances that extend spousal privileges to same-gender or unmarried couples, polyamory is still beyond the pale, although it is increasingly recognized as a valid choice. This may be because variations in relationship orientation are perceived as more of a threat to the established social order than are variations in sexual orientation.

WHO IS POLY?

For the rest of this chapter, we will use the word *poly* (the common prefix for *poly*gamy, *poly*gyny, *poly*andry, and *poly*fidelity) to refer to the relationship orientation of people who love and are open to being sexually intimate with more than one person at a time. This includes people who prefer to limit each individual sexual encounter to one person at a time even though they may have multiple partners as well as people who want to engage in group sex with their partners. It includes people who identify themselves as polyamorous as well as those who reject that label for one reason or another but whose behavior fits the definition of polyamory as presented in this book. It includes people who practice old-fashioned patriarchal polygamy (technically polygyny) where one man has more than one wife and polyandry where one woman has more than one husband. There is a strong trend in social science research these days not to impose labels or expectations on a target population, but because of the sensitive nature of coming out, in this discussion I think it's useful to include people who might not identify themselves as fitting into the poly world but who fit the definition I offered in chapter 1 of someone open to allowing love to determine the form of their relationships rather than deciding on one acceptable form and trying to force their relationships to fit into it.

For example, Amanda is a thirty-something-year-old woman reluctant to identify herself as poly because she's not sure whether she will want to be monogamous in the future, having chosen both monogamous and polyamorous relationships at different times in the past.

"Basically I'm asking myself now whether or not a poly lifestyle was a way for me to ease my way into a more lesbian lifestyle. I've considered myself bisexual for my entire adult life, having relationships with men but consistently fooling around with girls or just noticing how attracted I was to them. When I was twenty-two, I began a seven-year relationship with a man, one in which I never felt comfortable being monogamous partially because I was aware of how intensely I desired women. He and I were openly poly for the last four of the seven years. Our relationship ended when I chose to be monogamous with one of the women I was dating. This relationship with the woman ended two years later, but I still don't know whether I am poly or mono at heart or if it really has to do with the gender of the person I'm seeing or some other dynamics between me and the person I'm with. Regardless, I know that I am an open, loyal, and compassionate person, willing to work on my emotional stuff, and supportive of others working on theirs—all important qualities to nurture when in a polyamorous relationship."

There is a wide variety of lovestyles among people who are inclined toward same-gender partners, with some choosing monogamy, others preferring to have only anonymous encounters, and still others opting for open relationships or multiple committed relationships. Those with a poly orientation are equally diverse in their sexual orientations. They may be gay, straight, or bisexual, and they cover the entire middle ground between monogamy and promiscuity as well.

If we include everyone who's ever had two sexualoving partners during the same time period, even if they have not been open about it, as poly, we're talking about a lot of people. If we include people who constantly fantasize about other partners but don't act out their desires for fear of destroying their monogamous marriage, we're talking about even more people, so many that we can hardly call it a minority group. And if we include those practicing serial monogamy, which was called serial polygamy until the second half of the twentieth century, it's clearly a majority. Even if we only include people who have habitually had more than one lover at a time, whether single or married, there are a lot of polys out there. It's hard to know exactly how many, but current estimates for the United States put that number anywhere from half a million to 10 million people.

THE FALSE DICHOTOMY

People's sexual and relationship orientations don't always fit neatly into separate categories. For example, when I was in graduate school studying sexology, I was taught that on the homosexual–heterosexual dimension, there really isn't a dichotomy but, rather, a continuum. That is, on a scale of 1 to 10 where 1 is 100 percent heterosexual and 10 is 100 percent homosexual, most people will be somewhere in between the two extremes. People who are "somewhere in between" may—or may not—identify themselves as *bi*sexual. Until recently, most did not. I had never thought of myself as bisexual at the time, although it was clear to me when presented with the continuum concept that I fit somewhere in the middle.

To complicate matters even more, up until the late twentieth century, many professionals insisted that there was no such thing as a stable bisexual identity. That is, there was a belief that people who think they're bisexual are really in transition from the heterosexual pole to the homosexual pole

or vice versa. Only when relatively large numbers of self-identified bisexuals came forward saying that "gender is not the most important factor in
whom I love or don't love, and I consider myself to be bisexual whether I
happen to be with a same-gender partner or an opposite-gender partner or
none or both at any given time" was bisexuality acknowledged as a sexual
orientation. Bisexuals often remind us that our sexuality is more fluid than
we like to think and that we all have the potential to love people of both
genders. Some would rather not be confronted with this reminder.

Monogamy and polyamory may also be more of a continuum than a
dichotomy. Hardly anyone has only one sexual partner for their whole
lifetime, especially now that people are living twice as long they formerly
did. There is a big difference between being monogamous for twenty years
and being so for fifty. Hardly anyone has *never* had an exclusive relationship for at least a brief period. Most of us are somewhere in between.
And while some of those who are in between *are* in transition, others find
that having more than one committed sexualove relationship at a time is
what feels best to them. This does not preclude choosing to be with only
one partner for a period of time; it just means that there's no expectation
that the relationship will remain forever monogamous. Sometimes this in-
between group doesn't identify as poly simply because they've never met
or even heard of a person who has come out poly. This was certainly the
case with me until my early thirties, even though I had a long history of
being drawn to multiple partners.

David's experience also points to the importance of positive role models.
"I first heard of open and polyamorous relationships a few years ago when
I met several couples who enjoyed open relationships at a workshop. At
the time it made no sense to me, but later I decided to give it a try when
I was in love with a woman who only wanted to spend one and a half days
a week with me due to a busy work schedule. Rather than resenting her,
I told her that we either needed to break up, or I needed to have an additional relationship. Reluctantly, she said she would prefer me having other
lovers to ending the relationship, if I would practice safe sex. If I hadn't
met those open couples, I never would have thought of this, but it ended
up working out very well for me."

There's another strange thing about our efforts to categorize ourselves
and others. Not only do we try to make an *either/or* choice where a *both/
and* choice makes more sense, but we tend to put ourselves at the most
desirable pole and to put others at the less desirable pole even though

many of us are in the middle. This phenomenon is most obvious when we look at racial or ethnic identities. A person whose mother is white and whose father is black will be considered black in our culture. In Nazi Germany, a person with even a trace of Jewish blood was considered Jewish. However, many people of mixed blood "pass" as members of the dominant culture. Similarly, serial monogamists, who might more accurately be called serial polyamorists, pass as monogamists both to themselves and to society at large. And committed polys may reject the poly label because of its negative association with promiscuity in our culture. With models for responsible multipartner relationships still largely invisible, the concept of polyamory has often been seen as a male scam to avoid commitment or as evidence of nymphomania in a woman. Who would want to identify themselves with either of those stereotypes?

SEXUAL FLUIDITY

There is another factor to consider when looking at sexual and relationship orientations that has been called *sexual fluidity*. Psychologist Lisa Diamond hypothesizes that sexual identity is much more fluid in women than in men. She points out that most of the research on sexual orientation has been done exclusively on men and, after following a group of 100 young college women over a ten-year period, found that 60 percent of women who identified as lesbian at the beginning had some sort of sexual contact with men during the following ten years. Some changed their identity to bisexual or unlabeled, but even among lesbians who remained lesbian identified, 50 percent had some form of sexual contact with a man.[1]

Cardosa, Correia, and Capella have analyzed the relevance of the sexual fluidity concept for polyamory and conclude that "it seems that the data confirm what we've been arguing: the social setting of polyamory encourages sexual fluidity, and it is viewed as empowering and challenging, as having something to contribute to feminism as a social and political movement."[2]

If it's true, as Diamond suggests, that the emphasis on a fixed sexual identity is a masculine construct that is largely irrelevant for many women who place more importance on how they feel toward a particular individual regardless of gender, fluidity very likely applies to the relationship orientation of many women as well. The finding (discussed in chapter 2) that women are significantly more likely than men to give "falling in love" as a reason for chosing polyamory also supports Diamond's hypothesis. Amanda, whose story we considered previously, is a good example of a woman puzzled by the concept of a fixed identity that she has trouble locating herself within and who uses polyamory to try out different possibilities.

The feminine affinity for sexual fluidity would also go a long way toward explaining why virtually all the leadership in today's polyamory movement has come from women. The absence, up until now, of a theoretical framework that addresses the concept of sexual fluidity also explains why it's been so difficult for the "fluid" definition of polyamory that I put forward in the early 1990s emphasizing "letting love flow," whatever that ends up looking like, rather than forcing it into a predetermined form, to be taken seriously. Instead, definitions of polyamory that focus on a particular form for relationships or on the more obvious multipartner aspects of polyamory and that place polyamory in opposition to monogamy have most often been highlighted.

Cardosa, Correia, and Capella put it this way: "Let's begin with love then, with love's potential to destabilize sexual behaviors in women. The result, we posit, is that it becomes less and less relevant whether polyamory is truly (ontologically) about love or about sex, but that polyamory focuses on love, on feelings, as its main drive, as its discourse of election that it uses to convey meaning. And by doing so, it gains the power to directly address the questions and possibilities raised by sexual fluidity. . . . By defending and setting as its standard the possibility of non-exclusive relations and non-exclusive feelings, polyamory seems to provide a whole different background in which to live and try out different love configurations. And in a way, this contradicts to a point the effects of social and situational convergence either towards a heterosexual or a homosexual stable and normative identity."[3]

In other words, polyamory challenges the whole notion of normative sexual and relational identities, whether they be homosexual, heterosexual, monogamous, or nonmonogamous. In fact, this was the original intent of the polyamory movement, although it now is at risk for being seen as either a purely sexual diversion or a new normative standard that people may try to conform to, reject, or experience as a crisis of identity.

Consider the experience of Margaret, who came of age during the sexual revolution. Taking on a lesbian identity was a very deliberate radical and political action for her. She eagerly embraced the sexual fluidity concept when it was presented to her, saying, "I've been in a committed lesbian relationship for twenty-six years, and I have no intention of changing that. For the past few years I've been exploring polyamory and bisexuality, but I still consider myself a lesbian. It's very confusing."

Paradoxically, it's the very concept of sexual fluidity that, when incorporated into a polyamorous orientation, allows for the relative stability of a new paradigm flexible enough to include many diverse expressions of sexualove both within one individual at different times and across individuals—at least until the next paradigm shift comes around.

People often ask me if I still "believe" in polyamory or if I still want polyamorous relationships after all these years, and I always say that it depends on how they are defining polyamory. I can't imagine ever going back to a way of relating in which I give up the freedom to love whom I love or where someone else dictates whom I can and can't be sexual with. I can easily imagine choosing to focus with just one person whose presence I enjoy above all others. If this person were someone who could meet me on every level and who also chose to focus with me, I doubt very much that I'd have any interest in other sexual relationships. But to me, this continues to be polyamory because it's still fluid—the possibility is still there to openly have additional partners whether or not I actually do so.

WHERE HAVE ALL THE POLYS GONE?

You may be asking yourself, if there are so many polyamorous people that they might not even be in the minority, why are they not more visible? One reason is that so many polys have not come out—even to themselves. The concepts of coming out and being in the closet exist in the first place because a homosexual can easily present a public appearance of heterosexuality and go undetected unless she or he *chooses* to reveal him- or herself. However, in order to have a sexual encounter, a homosexual must come out at least to his or her prospective partner. In fact, the term *coming out* was originally used to refer to a first-time same-gender experience.

Someone who is nonmonogamous, however, can have sexual encounters without coming out to his or her partners as long as group sex is not involved. And the vast majority of polys rarely if ever engage in group sex. The polyamorous person is in somewhat the same situation as the bisexual who can, if he or she chooses, pass as straight with an opposite-gender lover and pass as gay or lesbian with a same-gender lover. And it is no coincidence that, until the past few decades, bisexuals have been pretty much invisible in both the heterosexual and the homosexual worlds. Sadly, one of the greatest fears that some bisexuals have about coming out is that it will be assumed that they're not monogamous.

Because polys can remain safely hidden while satisfying many sexual and emotional needs, they may lack the motivation to disclose their polyamorous feelings. They may also avoid coming out to themselves by telling themselves that they're trying to choose between several partners and have no intention of continuing to relate with more than one. It's easy for polys to imagine that they don't really *want* to have more than one lover at the same time; they're just having a hard time making up their mind—a very hard time. Or they may tell themselves and others that they don't really care for one of their partners; they're just there out of habit or obligation, or it's just a temporary fling.

Dana is twenty-one and a senior at the University of California. She doesn't consider herself polyamorous, but she often has more than one lover. This is how she sees it: "I'm not seriously involved with anyone at the moment. I have several 'friends with benefits,' but they're not real relationships. We're not thinking about getting married or anything; they're just good friends."

In my day, these kinds of relationships were called sexual friendships. Among baby boomers like myself, they have proven to sometimes be very enduring, emotionally intimate, and stable, outlasting many marriages or coexisting with them overtly or covertly. In fact, it's my observation that it is precisely because these friendships are not burdened with all the expectations and conditioning associated with marriage or with coupling up without benefit of marriage that they are often less volatile and more intimate than the relationship between spouses. Perhaps it will evolve differently with the younger generation, but clearly friends with benefits are somewhere in that middle ground between monogamous marriage and an anonymous one-night stand. Dana might not consider it polyamory, but it fits my definition.

It's natural for people to be reluctant to admit that what they want is something that's widely held to be immoral and indecent—not to mention impossible. But trying to repress, lie about, rationalize, or otherwise deny one's polyamorous nature can be very damaging to oneself, to loved ones, and the rest of the world. As we enter the twenty-first century, academic theorists, primarily in countries outside the United States, have begun to address the harmful impacts of heteronormative and mononormative social constructs and are attempting to introduce polyamory into the intellectual discourse on relationships, but mononormativity still prevails for the most part.

THE PRICE OF STAYING IN THE CLOSET

To go through life with the sense that one is guarding a dirty—and possibly dangerous—little secret is to go through life with ever-present feelings of isolation, alienation, and disharmony. Even if you limit your poly expression to the realm of fantasy and desire, you may experience a troubling sensation of not quite fitting in or being different from others in some mysterious, unknown way. The closeted person often feels as though he or she is from another planet. Depression, low self-esteem, and a lack of spontaneity are frequently problems.

Todd is a single man in his mid-fifties. He's been living with his partner Jane for two years, and they consider themselves married but decided against tying the knot legally because they've agreed to have an open relationship. Todd was raised in a fundamentalist Christian home where any sex outside of marriage, let alone multipartner sex, was a sure path to Hell. "I spent the first forty-five years of my life fighting my sexual urges. I married at twenty-one, mostly so I could have a sexual partner, but as it turned out, my wife hated sex and refused to even talk about it. Eventually, I fell in love with another woman and got a divorce so I could marry her. Our sex life was great until she got pregnant and completely lost interest in sex. I still loved her and didn't want to leave, and I didn't want to cheat, so I mostly fantasized about sex with other women and felt awful about myself. I was sure there was something wrong me and didn't dare discuss my desires with my wife—or anyone else for that matter. I was miserable. Finally, I got desperate enough that I went for an X-rated massage, which helped some, but I felt really guilty about it and was afraid my wife would find out. Then I saw an ad for a "dakini" that said she would teach me how to make sex spiritual. Well she did, and she also told me about polyamory. I fell in love with her, but I still loved my wife, and I just didn't know what to do. By this time, our son was two years

old, and I knew I couldn't abandon him, but I didn't want to give up my
dakini either. I was a mess."

It's hard to find compatible, like-minded partners without being up
front about who you are and what you want. And with so many polys in the
closet, it can be hard to locate compatible partners even if you are willing
to let others know that you're not monogamous. As with any suspect sub-
culture, the people most likely to come out initially include those who are
already so far out of the mainstream that they have little to lose by revealing themselves. This further distorts the already bizarre picture the public
has of polys as well as flooding an already small "gene pool" with potential
partners who are unsuitable for the average poly. Then there are people
who are still in the early stages of coming out to themselves and who may
get frightened and retreat to monogamy when faced with the prospect of
an actual poly relationship because they've never seen a successful one.
Consequently, some people give up and make a monogamous commitment
out of frustration rather than conviction.

The dearth of out-of-the-closet role models for creating a stable, legitimate poly lovestyle, combined with the perception of limited numbers of
potential partners, can create an atmosphere of pessimism, stuckness, and
scarcity. Very frequently, the first questions I'm asked by clients who come
to me for relationship coaching are, "Do you know anyone this is working
for?" Or, "Do you know any long-term open couples?" Even with more
people coming out, many still doubt that a healthy poly lovestyle is really
a possibility and have difficulty finding the support they need to overcome
the challenges inherent in any intimate relationship. Psychologist Geri
Weitzman discusses the difficulties polyamorous people have in finding
a therapist who will not pathologize them simply because they are poly
and cites a 2002 study that found that 38 percent of polyamorous people
who were in therapy chose not to even mention their poly lifestyle to their
therapist. Of those who did reveal it, 10 percent reported experiencing a
negative response. Even when a therapist was not judgmental, some clients
ending up using their paid session time to educate therapists who knew
nothing about polyamory.[4] Others will seek out a second professional to
supplement their regular therapist, who they perceive as unable to help
them manage an issue having to do with polyamory.

Beth was in a quandary about her marriage to a man who refused to
have sex with her. She consulted me to discuss the possibility of taking
on an outside lover. "Mitch won't even talk about sex with me; he just flat

out refuses to have anything to do with it, but he did say that it would be fine with him if I developed a sexual relationship with someone else. I was raised to believe that marriage meant being faithful to my husband, and the whole idea just seemed wrong to me, but then I met someone who's in an open relationship who I'm very attracted to. It seems like it might work. My therapist thinks I should leave Mitch, but we're so compatible in every other way, I don't want to divorce him, and he says he wants to stay married to me too."

When I asked what her therapist thought about her having sex with her new friend, Beth admitted that she didn't want to tell her therapist about this because she was too embarrassed and thought the therapist would disapprove. I urged her to bring all this to her regular therapist and told her I would continue working with her only if she first arranged for me to have a conversation with her therapist or if she terminated her other therapy and worked with me instead. Beth was surprised that I saw her effort to create a "secret therapy affair" instead of coming out to her therapist as an extension of the cultural pattern of infidelity. She was just doing what seemed normal to her, but that's what was creating her dilemma in the first place.

Some people do succeed in establishing satisfying nonmonogamous or extramarital relationships. While they are comfortably "out" to themselves and their partners, they still feel that they must hide their lovestyle from neighbors, employers, friends, and extended family. They may disguise a primary partner as a "roommate" or "housekeeper." They may camouflage a secondary partner as a "business associate" or "friend of the family." They may avoid restaurants and theaters where someone might recognize them. They may caution their children against discussing the extra partner with friends or teachers. They may simply keep quiet about their unconventional secret. These people may be less troubled than their solitary closet dwellers because they have each other for company. But they too pay a price for hiding out and often feel isolated and afraid of being discovered.

Ricky is a twenty-year-old college student who was raised in a polyamorous household. He recalls, "I wasn't really aware of my parents' sex life when I was a child. I just saw the other adults who were around as friends. That changed when I got older and became interested in sex. When I was about thirteen, my mother told me Social Services had the power to come into our house and take me away, so I shouldn't let anybody know that she had more than one partner. I felt scared. I remember feeling confused and angry too. Why? Why would somebody take me out of my home? I felt totally safe and happy there."

Hiding your polyamorous lifestyle from your children, particularly as they get older, and pretending to endorse monogamy doesn't work very well either, as they are likely to reflect the judgments of the mononormative culture they've been raised in when they accidentally discover Mom or Dad has a secret life. Those who are actively nonmonogamous without coming out to their lovers, spouses, and children may hide their pain and feelings of worthlessness under the excitement of intrigue and illicit adventure. But one lie—or omission—leads to another, and pretty soon they're lying all the time. Leading a double life can be stressful as well as effectively limiting deep intimacy with others. When they're found out, they not only hurt the ones they love but also condition their partners to associate nonmonogamy with the betrayal of trust, a confusion from which they may never recover.

People who choose not to come out, even with admirable motivations, add their weight to the legacy of deceit and infidelity that polys everywhere must contend with and strengthen the bad reputation and mononormative illusion that may have led them to stay in the closet in the first place. Everyone is disempowered by the failure to stand up and be counted, just as all can be empowered by the courage of those able and willing to take the risk of coming out.

However, coming out can come with a price. In the past, admitting to nonmonogamy, not to mention advocating it, could be life threatening or lead to prosecution as a sex offender. Fortunately, these dramatic outcomes are no longer common. But for people whose effectiveness in the world would be compromised by coming out poly, it may be wiser to keep their private lives private from all but their most intimate friends and family. Often, people's fears are greater than the reality, but, as one professional told me, "The day polyamorists are treated socially and professionally as true equals of monogamists is the day I will come out."

THE OUTCOMES OF COMING OUT

The prejudice against polyamory can extend to those who merely choose to research it. Perhaps this accounts in part for the lack of academic attention given to polyamory. One bold young social scientist who chose to make polyamory the topic of her doctoral research reports that "defending my dissertation was the worst day of my life so far. One committee member verbally attacked me and didn't want to accept the research for reasons which would not have arisen with another topic. My chair was aghast at the outburst. The whole committee was open-mouthed shocked about the things this woman said to me."

Other researchers, particularly those who try to combine activism with academia, find that their colleagues don't take their work seriously. Worse yet, if they risk coming out, they are sometimes reprimanded for violating propriety. One faculty member confided, "One of the hardest things I've ever done was to go back and lecture my students after having been told off for 'bringing the institution into disrepute' and also told that other members of staff would no longer be able to look me in the eye."

Unfortunately, even the most conservative polyamorist can be portrayed as a slut by journalists seeking a sensationalist story, and one television producer who frequently called me desperately seeking out-of-the-closet polyamorous families for a popular talk show told me that she always tried to schedule a polyamory topic during "sweeps week" because it was a sure way to increase ratings.

Another professional woman who took the risk of coming out says that it "led to a big explosion for me personally and professionally, which I didn't expect at all. I don't regret it because I care passionately about these issues and am politically committed to outness. But it was very hard to deal with for all kinds of reasons. Particularly, it was hard to know that lots of people who didn't even know me had strong, sometimes negative opinions about me. I still have a way to go in terms of processing some of what I've been through."

As we've seen in other chapters, coming out can also have negative consequences for people in certain professions who have lost their livelihoods and for parents who've lost custody of their children. Even when custody has not been an issue, children can be ostracized by peers or by friends' parents who don't want their own child to visit a polyamorous home or can be pathologized by teachers, counselors, or neighbors who project their own fears onto the children.

For people in less sensitive occupations that involve little contact with the public or that tend to be tolerant of diversity, such as the computer and software industries, reactions can be more varied and more personal with less potential to adversely affect careers. One computer programmer who came out at work says that his coworkers' reactions "ran the whole gamut. Some were fascinated in a sensationalistic way, others were personally interested and wanted to have a drink after work and talk about it, some were freaked out—I think those may have been people who'd experienced infidelity. But there were absolutely no negative consequences as far as my job goes."

Because of the potential for negative reactions, some polyamorous people have decided to change careers or relocate to less conservative areas. In today's global village, with so many people changing jobs and geography, such shifts can occur for many other reasons, but they can still be disruptive, particularly for children and extended families. Interestingly enough, most people I've spoken to who've come out to parents and other relatives report that their families have been very accepting of additional partners.

There are always exceptions, but in general the earlier in life one begins one's coming-out process, the easier it will be. The younger you are, the less likely you are to have created structures in your life that will have to be dismantled as a result of coming out. However, most people go through developmental crises throughout their adult lives. A divorce, a career change, a spiritual awakening, the death of a loved one, an "empty nest," or retirement are all opportunities to consider embracing a new relationship orientation.

Not surprisingly, the context in which people are most likely to experience painful rejection is coming out to a spouse or other intimate partner who has been promised monogamy. You can be met with a hostile or indignant response simply to the news that you have polyamorous desires or fantasies, even without any violations of a monogamous commitment or effort to renegotiate a monogamous agreement. If this is the case, an open-minded therapist can often be invaluable in creating safety and support for both partners to communicate their fears and reexamine their motivations and bottom lines.

Because of the potential for negative impacts of coming out, everyone needs to evaluate the risks and benefits of coming out for themselves in their particular situation. For many people, the benefits of coming out, at least to yourself and those closest to you, far outweigh the risks. But endangering whatever is precious to you is not something to take lightly, and sacrificing your own well-being to make a statement may be unwise. At the same time, I feel strongly that one of the best gifts a person can give him- or herself is the permission to authentically be who he or she is. Permission to *be* who you are doesn't mean giving yourself license to *do* anything at all, as people sometimes fear. Rather, it's a way to become more conscious about what you want and why and so become better equipped to find a balance between pleasing only yourself and pleasing everyone but yourself. Accepting yourself as a polyamorous person is an important part of the larger process of self-differentiation and integration. It liberates you from having to hide an important part of yourself, and hiding tends to slow down or even stop the whole growth process. Worse yet, if you deny your poly nature, you may end up projecting it outside yourself and see sex-crazed demons under every rock that you then try to restrain and control. Or you can unconsciously transform your unused sexualoving potential into hatred and aggression.

Coming to terms with your relationship orientation is an essential—and often neglected—part of growing up and becoming a mature human being. Not only does it contribute to your personal well-being, but it increases your capacity to share intimacy with others as well. Coming out makes it *possible* to establish ethical and stable relationships. It allows you to be more open and honest with everyone you know because you no longer have to censor yourself to prevent an inadvertent slip.

Each person who comes out poly increases the likelihood that others will become aware of their own poly identity and feel safe disclosing it. The more people come out, the more easily others will be able to find and support each other. The more people take the risk of being openly and responsibly polyamorous, the sooner the confusion between patriarchal polygamy, uncommitted promiscuity, and committed nonmonogamous relationships will be clarified and the sooner mononormative thinking will give way to greater acceptance of diversity. When a critical mass of polyamorous people have come out, the outmoded paradigm of sexualove as a scarce and jealously guarded resource will shift. A new paradigm will emerge in which sexualove is an abundant and renewable gift to be responsibly shared at will.

HOW TO COME OUT

A good way to begin the coming-out process is by reviewing relevant personal history. Asking these questions will help clarify the extent to which a person identifies as polyamorous and how he or she feels about it:

Have you ever had more than one lover or boyfriend or girlfriend at a time?

Have you heard of polyamory? What does it mean to you?

Do you consider yourself polyamorous?

How do you feel about polyamory?

Have you ever told anyone you were nonmonogamous?

If yes, what exactly did you say, and how did they respond? Who else have you told? Why?

When did you first meet someone who was poly?

Next, review the people who are either partners or potential partners and ask the following questions:

How honest have I been about my romantic and sexual desires, encounters, fantasies, and conflicts with person x, y, and z? (don't forget to include yourself)

How honest do I want to be with person x, y, and z?

How risky does it feel to be more honest with person x, y, and z?

If it becomes clear that a person is not monogamous but feels that it's too risky to let *anyone* know that one is poly, one probably still feels that he or she is doing something wrong. My recommendation would be to find a support group or an open-minded therapist to explore some of these issues. If this is not possible, starting a journal where private feelings and experiences can be recorded is a good alternative. Talking to strangers or new acquaintances can also provide an opportunity to try being more honest with people where there is little risk involved.

Twenty-five years ago, following the publication of my first book on polyamory, television producers started calling me with requests to appear on various talk shows. They usually wanted me to bring a husband or lover or three, and they often asked me to help them find other polyamorous families to fill out the show. I found that my own and others' coming-out issues were quickly elicited by the prospect of discussing our relationships on national television. In those days, it took a very confident or very naive person to expose their intimate lives to television hosts and audiences who were often critical, judgmental, and downright hostile.

While most people found this prospect too daunting to seriously consider doing it, thinking and talking about it turned out to be an excellent window into coming-out issues. I created the following exercise for people attending my seminars on polyamory and called it "Shine the Light of Television into Your Closet." Imagine that you've just received a phone call from the producers of a national talk show. They want to know if you'll appear as a guest to talk about your nonmonogamous lovestyle. "And could you bring any of your lovers with you?" they ask. You take a deep breath and tell them you'll have to think about it. They say they'll get back to you in a few days.

Now ask yourself the following questions: What is your greatest fear about appearing on this talk show? What questions might be asked that you wouldn't want to answer on national television? What would be hard to explain? What might you feel embarrassed or ashamed about? What would you be most proud of? Who would or would not be willing to accompany you? Who would you be afraid would see you? What would you not want them to find out about you? What consequences (negative or positive) might result from your appearance on the show?

Try to write down at least some of your answers. Now ask yourself the following: What would have to change in your life for you to feel comfortable appearing on this TV show? What would be the easiest to change? The hardest?

Another good coming-out exercise is to write a coming-out letter. Here is one suggested format. Choose someone from your cast of characters to whom you would like to but have not yet come out. If possible, choose a pivotal person, such as a lover, parent, or close friend. Then begin by telling this person about your positive feelings toward him or her. Express how much you value your relationship with him or her and offer appreciation for his or her contributions to your life. If you're writing to someone whom you have mixed feelings toward or who you feel has wronged you or misunderstood you in the past, such as a parent or ex-spouse, be careful not to blame or judge him or her for what he or she has done. Instead, tell him or her about the hurt that you've felt and how you've tried to protect yourself from feeling that hurt. Then share whatever you can about being nonmonogamous and proud. If you know that the person you're writing to is an ardent monogamist, be sure to emphasize that you respect his or her choices and you'd like him or her to respect yours. If you feel ready to take the risk, mail the letter. If you don't, ask yourself this: What might I gain from sharing this letter? What might I lose?

WHEN SOMEONE YOU KNOW COMES OUT POLY

If someone you know tells you that he or she is poly, it's best to be honest about your response, whatever that may be. Using "I" statements is a good way to frankly make your feelings known without judging or attacking. For example, you could say, "I notice that I felt anxious when you said you have another partner." Or, "I'm feeling angry you didn't tell me this before." Or, "I'm so relieved! I was wondering if you would reject me if I told you that I've never been monogamous." If you're curious and want to hear more about it or if you have relevant experiences of your own, that can be part of the conversation too, but it's a good idea to check in with yourself and see if there are any unexpressed emotional reactions first. On the other hand, it's fine to set your own boundaries and say that you need some time to process what you've heard and that you don't want to discuss it just yet.

Remember that whomever you're talking with may be nervous or even terrified about how you'll react, especially if it's someone close to you. They may interpret a remark such as "That explains a lot" in a negative way even if you didn't mean it as a judgment. Starting with an appreciation, such as "Thank you for trusting me with this information" or "I'm happy we're getting to know each other better," can be a good way to offer reassurance that you're not planning an attack.

POLYAMORY AND THE LAW

While many Middle Eastern, Asian, and African nations still permit men to marry more than one woman, Western countries consider a legal marriage to more than one person at a time to constitute the crime of bigamy (although exceptions are made in some countries for immigrants from polygamous cultures). In North America, most of the twenty-first-century legal action affecting polys seems to be surfacing in Canada rather than the United States. In 2005, the Canadian government appointed a commission to investigate the status of immigrant women and children who came to Canada as part of polygamous families. Several papers were published, but no legal changes were enacted.

Muslims have long argued that plural marriage provides more protection to women than the Western custom of keeping mistresses. Betsy's story illustrates the veracity of the Muslim position as well as the reality that legal protections can always be circumvented. Betsy, an attractive redhead in her late forties, has been in relationship with Terry, who's in his late fifties, for over ten years. Both are divorced with grown children from their previous marriages. They lived together briefly earlier on, but

Terry prefers to maintain separate households although his huge estate is usually half empty. He gives Betsy a monthly allowance and pays for their frequent vacations as well as other "extras" that she wouldn't be able to afford on her part-time yoga teacher salary. Betsy, who has identified as bisexual and nonmonogamous since she was a teenager, is challenged by Terry's refusal to openly communicate about his other girlfriends. "I don't know what he expects me to think when I find another woman's lingerie in his closet," she says. "It's obvious there's another woman, but he refuses to discuss it. It annoys me that he won't be honest with me, but otherwise it's not a problem, except when I feel he's neglecting me, which does happen from time to time. Like any relationship, ours ebbs and flows, but because he won't tell me what's going on with him, I never know if it's a new woman or if his family is making more demands on him or he just needs some downtime."

Betsy usually responds to Terry's occasional distancing by deciding to find another partner who will be more consistently available and willing to talk honestly about other love interests, but she's never found anyone she likes better than Terry. Terry objects to her having other lovers, but Betsy always argues that if he can do it, she can too. Once he threatened to cut off her allowance but relented when she refused to give in. Despite these difficulties, Betsy and Terry continue to keep choosing each other. There are no legal obstacles to their getting married, but Terry prefers to keep Betsy in the mistress role. Betsy worries that without any legal guarantees, she won't be provided for as a wife would be if Terry were to die before her but shrugs and says, "It's about love, not money."

In the United States, renegade Mormons who never relinquished their polygamous customs periodically surface and sometimes face legal action for tax evasion or child abuse and statutory rape when underage wives are involved but otherwise continue to live undisturbed as they always have. But in British Columbia, Canada, where a case against renegade Mormon polygamists was dismissed on a technicality in 2009, a ruling is being sought as to whether Canadian laws prohibiting polygamy are legal.

The poly community is following this case closely because it could set a precedent one way or the other not only on plural marriage but also on the ability of more than two polyamorous people to live together even if they don't call it a marriage. The same law that prohibits patriarchal polygamy also makes it a crime, punishable by five years in prison, to conduct—or even attend—a ceremony sanctioning a multipartner union even if there is no attempt at a legal marriage. Although parts of this nearly forgotten nineteenth-century law are in violation of Canada's newer Charter of Rights and Freedoms, the desire to punish the allegedly child and woman–abusing Mormon polygamist cult leaders seems to be overriding concerns about freedom—but not in the Canadian polyamory community, where organizers are seeking "intervenors" (polyamorous people willing to swear an affidavit in court) to testify that the nineteenth-century law is unconstitutional and should be struck down.

While it seems unlikely that the law will be used to prosecute polyamorists who are otherwise good citizens, gay activists warn that test cases do matter. There are many outmoded laws still on the books in countries all over the globe. In the United States, as in most places, such laws are rarely enforced, but their presence can add an additional layer of fear, guilt, and shame that discourages people from coming out.

The Canadian polyamory community recognizes that this high-profile legal case presents an opportunity to educate people about the difference between patriarchal polygamy and polyamory as well as the rather remote possibility of legalizing group marriage in Canada, but in order to do so, they need to find credible intervenors giving details of their loving, committed, consensual live-in relationships involving more than two adults and willing to have their names, addresses, and other information made public and possibly reported on in the newspapers. Perhaps changing an antiquated law is a better reason to come out than entertaining television viewers, but there is no way around the coming-out challenges associated with volunteering for this task.

I don't think the question has ever been posed to the poly community in a systematic way, but, while 72 percent of the poly people surveyed by *Loving More* magazine said that they supported "multiple marriage," in my experience the reality is that the vast majority of polyamorous people don't want to be married—legally or not—to more than one person at a time. Only 3 percent of those surveyed indicated that they were in a group marriage, and more than half were not married at all. This is a reflection primarily of the greater popularity of couple-oriented open marriage within the poly community but also the overall increase in unmarried but cohabiting couples in society at large as well as the sentiment that "the state" has no business involving itself in people's private lives.

However, some people feel that legalizing group marriage would be one way to demonstrate that polyamory has the "social seal of approval" as well as providing legal rights to health care, insurance, housing, tax benefits, child custody, inheritance, and other privileges normally associated with marriage. In a practical sense, all these legal considerations can be addressed without benefit of a marriage contract, either through a corporate vehicle or by individual contracts. Valerie White, a polyamorous attorney who directs the Sexual Freedom Legal Defense and Education Fund, advises polyamorous partners on how to protect themselves within the existing legal framework. Although the center does provide some pro bono counsel, especially for poly parents with custody issues, leaving it to the individual to draft his or her own customized contracts means that polys who are low income and/or less educated have less access to legal protection.

Six states in the United States now recognize same-gender marriage, as do some European countries. Many municipalities have adopted "domestic partners" regulations that allow any two people who share a domicile and income share, for a specified length of time, access to the same benefits given to spouses, but resistance to allowing more than two domestic partners to register together seems just as high as expanding the definition of marriage to include polyamorous as well as same-gender unions. Tampering with the current "one man, one woman" definition of marriage triggers incredibly strong emotional reactions, particularly among conservative Christians, who have demonstrated political clout well beyond their numbers. However, polls show that age is strongly related to people's positions on marriage, and as the twenty-first century progresses, marriage laws may well come up for review, and some poly activists are preparing for this eventuality.

Sina Pichler is a graduate student at the University of Vienna in Austria, where she is conducting research on polyamory for her thesis. She's been closely following the ongoing discussion among poly activists concerning legalizing polyamorous marriage. Many feel that new marital legislation should be globalized rather than left to states or nations in keeping with the spirit of today's global village. Some of the debate centers on the relative merits of allowing a form of marriage that she calls "all-with-all," in which three or more people are joined together at the same time within a single marriage, versus "dyadic networks," in which existing laws against bigamy are revised so that people can be concurrently married more than once, provided that each new marriage is preceded by notification to existing spouse(s) of the pending new marriage.

Pichler favors the "dyad network" version of plural marriage on the grounds that it minimizes changes to the existing system while providing access to marriage for a variety of poly families, including those situations that the all-with-all model doesn't address. She points out that in most multiple-partner relationships, all partners don't marry at once, and in the "V" or "N" structures, all the partners may not even be connected to each other. (In a V, Susie may be "married" to Hank and Isaac, but Isaac is not "married" to Hank. In an N, Susie may be "married" to Hank and Isaac, and then Isaac may "marry" Chris.) The dyad network also has advantages in the event of divorce, where one dyad can split up while leaving the rest of the connections intact.

In addition, Pichler argues that the all-with-all model is too limiting since its size cannot exceed the number of individuals who have a "meeting of mind." The molecular-building-block nature of the dyad network means that its size is virtually unlimited. In theory, "every adult on earth" could be joined together into one enormous dyadic network.

I doubt that the full vision will be implemented anytime soon, but it's a good example of the creative thinking of polyamorous people. Perhaps legalizing a simple triadic marriage, even if it includes two same-gender partners, would be the conservative way to go.

9

CROSS-CULTURAL PERSPECTIVES

I first realized just how international polyamory was becoming when I offered a seminar in Greece in the fall of 2003. Around this time I also started getting phone calls from British and French television producers who were hoping I could find them some American polyamorous families willing to appear in their documentary projects. The occasional Brit or European had been making the long transatlantic flight to attend various workshops I facilitated for years, but offering a weeklong seminar on the European continent created a mini United Nations. Half the group was made up of Americans and Canadians, but a total of twelve nationalities were represented—a lot considering that we had fewer than twenty participants. We had an Italian professor from Rome, an Indian stockbroker from Bombay, a British computer programmer, an Egyptian scientist, a French musician, an Iranian doctor, and a Catholic couple from the Netherlands who had left their two children at home in the care of another couple with whom they were intimate.

Instead of holding the seminar at the Findhorn-inspired retreat center of Kalikos in the north of Greece as planned, a last-minute venue change landed us on the island of Lesvos in a lovely villa overlooking the Aegean Sea and a short walk from an ancient bathhouse where hot springs bubbled into a cavelike enclosure over a stone soaking pool as well as into the pebbly seashore outside. Lesvos, the birthplace of the famous bisexual, polyamorous fifth-century B.C. poet Sappho, turned out to be the perfect place to begin my exploration of polyamory around the world. Sappho is revered by lesbians the world over, and her home (sometimes spelled "Lesbos") has even lent its name to identify women who love women and is a major pilgrimage site for lesbians today. While much of Sappho's exquisite poetry and the details of her life have been lost, she could just as easily be seen as an illustrious ancestor for polys as for lesbians since she apparently had relationships with both genders. In any case, the ancient Greeks were a sex-positive people well into recorded history, as is evident from classical-era art and matriarchal myth, and despite the influence of the Greek Orthodox Church, this can be felt even now in the relaxed attitudes toward nudity and exuberant enjoyment of life still evident there today.

The 2003 seminar became my initiation to the European continent, and while I have since traveled extensively throughout Asia, India, and Turkey, I've still not experienced much of Europe, the United Kingdom, Africa, or Australia firsthand. However, people from all over the world have migrated to the San Francisco Bay Area, long a magnet for social and cultural experimentation, where I lived, worked, and played for several decades. The Internet has also helped the culture of polyamory to spread worldwide. Facebook's Polyamory Europe Group lists upcoming polyamory meetings in Dublin, Helsinki, Paris, London, Turku, Barcelona, and Girona (Spain), and India has its own separate Facebook group.

One of the many paradoxes of polyamory is that while today's polyamory movement clearly arose in the United States and while the United States gave birth to many nineteenth-century communities that enthusiastically explored nonmonogamous relationships, not to mention countless twentieth-century hippie communes, all the major openly polyamorous communities of the twenty-first century are outside the United States to the best of my knowledge. The whole concept of polyamorous communities is a tricky one for a variety of reasons. For example, one of the best-known intentional communities in the world was started by a polyamorous triad masquerading as a couple and their good friend. This community continues to be a model and inspiration for many, although it has never been able to do very well with integrating sexuality into its philosophy, and most of its members have no idea of the truth about its origins.

Other communities, such as ZEGG in Germany (discussed later in this chapter), reject the label "polyamory" but put a lot of focus on *freie Liebe*, or "free love," as part of a larger vision for ecological living. Meanwhile,

American polys tend to avoid the language of free love because of its association with promiscuity in the days of the sexual revolution. The notoriously individualistic Americans generally prefer open couples or intimate networks to group marriages or communal living, but there are long-standing intentional communities in the United States where polyamory has been quietly practiced, openly or closeted, along with old-fashioned infidelity on occasion amidst considerable drama and processing.

Another noteworthy difference between North American and continental mores is that even though a probable majority of Americans who call themselves monogamous are not sexually exclusive, Americans take monogamy much more seriously than Europeans. While much of the civilized world espouses monogamy but takes discrete affairs for granted, Americans tend to believe that extramarital sex is wrong and are prone to tremendous guilt and shame when they fail to honor their monogamous commitments. Perhaps polyamory's appeal to Americans—and Australians as well—is that in these cultures, a combination of sexual repression, boring sex, and the taboo on extramarital sex as a solution to marital monotony create an unmet need for a pragmatic, direct, egalitarian means of spicing up a marriage. In Europe and the United Kingdom, polyamory seems more of interest to those with a political bent who appreciate the anarchistic appeal of free love as advocated by Emma Goldman and who are as moved by the ecological considerations and the moral high ground as juicy sex. Europeans who want more or different sex simply have an affair. Of course, plenty of American couples have affairs too, or they turn to swinging for sexual variety but sometimes end up falling in love with their sexual playmates.

I expanded into an international perspective relatively late in life, but my perceptions are similar to those of best-selling author Esther Perel, a New York couples therapist who grew up in Europe and specializes in cross-cultural issues. Perel observes that "egalitarianism, directness, and pragmatism are entrenched in American culture and inevitably influence the way we think about and experience love and sex. Latin Americans' and Europeans' attitudes toward love, on the other hand, tend to reflect other cultural values, and are more likely to embody the dynamics of seduction, the focus on sensuality, and the idea of complementarity (i.e., being different but equal) rather than absolute sameness. . . . Some of America's best features—the belief in democracy, equality, consensus-building, compromise, fairness, and mutual tolerance—can, when carried too punctiliously into the bedroom, result in very boring sex. Sexual desire and good citizenship don't play by the same rules."[1]

With this prelude, let's move on to consider the experiences of polyamorous people around the world. What I've observed as I've led seminars and coached partners and families in over a dozen different countries is that the issues people are struggling with in their relationships and the ways in which their own conditioning and biology come into conflict are remarkably similar everywhere. At the same time, each nationality has a unique flavor and history that gives their polyamorous forays a distinctive quality. A thorough discussion of polyamory in every country or even on every continent is beyond the scope of this chapter. What follows is an overview from selected countries around the world where I have spent the most time or have found people most attracted to polyamory.

CHINA

In 2008, I traveled to mainland China and Hong Kong for the first time. My older daughter and her family were living in Beijing, and I was to meet with a sociology professor at the Chinese Academy of Social Sciences who intended to publish Sonia Song's Chinese translation of my book *Polyamory: The New Love without Limits* as part of a series on human sexuality. As it turned out, the printing was delayed first by an earthquake, then by the Olympics, and then by the government censors, who apparently found polyamory an inappropriate subject at the time, although they had permitted publication of books on homosexuality and bisexuality. China, like the United States, is a vast country that now encompasses many ethnic minorities, including a sizable population of Muslims, in addition to dominant Han Chinese. Beijing, where I spent most of my time, is known as a conservative, traditional city relative to cosmopolitan Shanghai, which has welcomed foreign travelers for centuries. Hong Kong, despite long years of rule by the British, is perhaps more traditionally Chinese than mainland China in certain ways, and it was far easier for me to communicate with people there because so many people speak English, a British legacy I welcomed.

Prior to the Communist Revolution in China, which resulted in a ban on polygamy in 1953, there was a long tradition of patriarchal polygamy, with affluent men routinely having multiple wives. After the rise of Confucianism around the first century A.D., technically only one woman was the official wife, and the rest were called concubines. In the case of royalty, women had multiple lovers as well in the distant past, as discussed in chapter 10. The old Chinese system was very hierarchical with wives and concubines having specific status and legal rights and all knowing their "place." Nevertheless, a young and ambitious concubine sometimes managed to win the affections of a powerful man and gain privileges that were not rightfully hers. In Hong Kong, where polygyny was not banned until 1971, there are many adults who were raised in these families with one legal wife and several concubines. Many sources say that the tradition continues, even though concubines are no longer legally recognized and so have no property rights.

Richard, who is now in his late fifties, is the oldest son of Li Yan and Zhao Song. Li Yan was once the number two "wife," of Wang Jing. Wang Jing had three children with Li Yan and had children with his other three wives as well. All lived harmoniously in a large family compound. When Wang Jing died, Li Yan married Wang Jing's business partner Zhao Song, with whom she had four more children. Richard considers all of Wang Jing's children to be his brothers and sisters, even those with a different mother. Together they make up a large and close-knit extended family.

Richard* is recently engaged to Kate, a British woman who originally came to Hong Kong twenty years ago with her former husband. Richard and Kate are a cosmopolitan professional couple who could be at home anywhere in the world. Richard's ex-wife, Susan, who is also British, returned to London with their three children after their divorce four years ago. Richard visits at their home several times a year to be with his children and participate in Susan's family gatherings. This seems quite natural to Richard, perhaps because of his own polygamous upbringing, but Kate has doubts about his staying at Susan's home, even though Richard insists it's just practical and not sexual. "I liked the idea in theory," says Kate, "but found it harder to live with, especially when I was visiting my parents just across town. I felt like a mistress! This year we're going back together for two weeks, and he will stay with me and visit them." Kate says that she and Richard are happily monogamous at the moment, but they've discussed polyamory as an option somewhere down the line. "We'd consider taking

---

*It is common among Hong Kong Chinese, especially those born after World War II, to have English nicknames by which they identify themselves, at least when interacting with English-speaking people.

on another wife if someone turned up who was attractive to both of us, but we're not looking," says Kate.

Don also grew up in Hong Kong and is about ten years younger than Richard. His mother was a concubine of Zhang Guo Qiang, a wealthy and powerful businessman, but unlike Richard's big, happy clan, Don's family life was quite traumatic for him. "My father's number one wife had no sons, only daughters. When I was born, my birth mother handed me over to the number one wife, and I never saw her again, nor did my father. Mom Mei, as I called her, and her daughters were abusive to me all through my childhood. Even today, the daughters' husbands, my brothers-in-law, are my enemies. They are envious. As the only son of my father, I am receiving what they feel should be theirs."

Don consulted me because he wanted to learn more about polyamory after his Singapore-raised Chinese ex-wife, Denise, proclaimed herself polyamorous and divorced him. "I'm still very close friends with Denise and her boyfriend Gary," he told me. "No one will ever take her place in my heart. We are no longer sexual, although we sometimes spend the night together, and recently Denise has asked to be lovers again. My girlfriend, Ann, is very unhappy about my continuing friendship with Denise. Ann wants me to marry her and threatens to leave me if I won't, but I just don't trust her. I'm afraid she will take my money and leave me for another man." Don is a sensitive and empathic man who realizes that Ann carries the legacy of generations of Chinese women who were lovers to Chinese men but denied their rightful place in the family. After several sessions with me, he realized that he still holds on to the hope of getting back together with Denise but doesn't think he can overcome his jealousy with Gary or the childhood wounds that have left him distrustful of women and afraid of their anger. Meanwhile, Ann has discovered that by taking on another lover, she can push Don to offer her marriage even though he still feels conflicted about this. "I love her, and I don't want to lose her, but I'm afraid she is manipulating me. And she feels the same way about me," he moans. "Polyamory may offer you some compelling reasons to heal the past," I tell him, "but I can't recommend it to you. You're moving way too fast! Slow down. Take one piece at a time and don't allow yourself to be pulled on to the next one until you're ready, or you're in for some big dramas. It's admirable to want to heal legions of Chinese women, including even your own dead mother, but let's start with you first!"

It's my impression that the Chinese have an odd combination of idealism, shrewdness, innocence, and pragmatism. Whether through Chinese tradition or communism, they have often been taught to put others' needs ahead of their own. Although the social codes can be rigid, especially in regard to family obligations, they tend to be generally more relaxed about bodily functions and accept sexuality as a natural part of life as long as it follows the rules. I spoke with one bright young Hong Kong Chinese woman who had attended boarding school in England and was disowned by her mother after disclosing that she'd had sex with her boyfriend without benefit of marriage. Another sought my help to help create a satisfying sexual relationship with her husband after pretending to be orgasmic to entice him into marriage. Like many American men, he was eager to please her but simply didn't know how, and she was afraid to appear too experienced.

Beijing sociologist Li Yin He estimates that over 10 million women in mainland China are married to homosexuals who marry and have children to fulfill family expectations even though they know they are gay.[2] To further complicate things, the "one-child" policy instituted to control China's burgeoning population has had the unanticipated side effect of creating a scarcity of single women of marriageable age, as many couples in the previous generation made sure that if they could only have one child, it would be a son. One practical solution to the resulting gender imbalance would be to institute polyandry, but this may be a bit too practical even for the post–Cultural Revolution Chinese and perhaps a little too Tibetan as well, with Tibet's history of allowing women multiple husbands.

In mainland China, the Cultural Revolution left in its wake a moral vacuum. Chairman Mao's philosophy is now suspect, and meanwhile centuries-old traditions of Taoism and Tibetan Buddhism were scorned and temples turned into factories. Only a few remnants exist from which to piece together the past. Prior to the Communist Revolution in China, Tibetan lamas were highly influential advisers to the emperors. Both the Taoists and the Tibetan Buddhists are known for their sophisticated and explicit teachings on sexual union as a means of achieving greater health, happiness, and spiritual awareness. Today, many westerners have a greater understanding of these traditions than the average Chinese, who is interested more in emulating the material success of Americans than in resurrecting the spiritual traditions of an earlier era. Young people are confused about what constitutes ethical and realistic sexual mores.

As a result of all these factors, I believe that China is ripe for polyamory. When the conflicts between the age-old tradition of polygamy for (wealthy) men only, the modern ideal of equal rights for women, and Christian influences toward sexual repression are resolved, polyamory may well be recognized as a valid option for preserving the all-important extended family. This is important in China, where many of the government-sponsored social supports and health care options we take for granted even in the proudly capitalist United States are not part of the infrastructure.

Sonia Song, who we first met in chapter 2, came from Beijing to Berkeley, California, in 1987 to study law. She found in polyamory a way to reconcile her ideals with her personal needs for sexual expression, loving support, and extended family. Inspired by the freedom and democracy she saw in the United States, she was also appalled by the crime, violence, and wastefulness and disheartened by the loneliness, isolation, and alienation she felt. Noting that placing the common good above the self is a core value both in Western democracy and in Eastern communism, she didn't hesitate to bring this value into her intimate relationships once given the chance. In her touching memoir *Donkey Baby*, she writes that after arriving in the United States, she still yearned for the sense of community that she had learned in the Beihai kindergarten in Beijing, where food, clothes, toys, friends, and caretakers were all shared. Sonia explored the Christian religion but found that its brand of love didn't suit her. "I wanted it to be a matter of choice—a voluntary communion with those I feel most closely connected to, freely given from my own heart, not dictated by conformity, convention, or compulsion. . . . I wanted to keep the freedom I had found in the West, and I wanted to regain the commitment to a greater good that I had learned in the East. . . . For me, love as an abstraction is not enough. Love that I feel on a personal level is precious. Can I feel a personal love for one human being? Yes. More than one? Yes. If divine love is inclusive, why should human love be exclusive? Why not share love?"[3]

Before her introduction to polyamory, Sonia reports that "I used to have dysfunctional relationships—marriage without love, love without sex, sex without love—all messed up." Sonia met her future husband at a polyamorous gathering. He was almost eighty at the time, nearly forty years older than herself, and was a retired sociology professor who had spent a lifetime exploring alternative ways to love. Sonia was attracted emotionally, spiritually, and intellectually and was delighted to find they were sexually compatible as well. They soon rented a house together, and her son came to live with them. Sonia had two other lovers she'd met at a polyamorous event. One of the lovers was not respectful of her new primary relationship, but her new partner was wise enough to allow her the freedom to make her own choices, and eventually she chose to discontinue the other relationship. The intimacy with the other secondary continued, with both men enjoying friendship with each other as well as with Sonia. After Don's death, Sonia was devastated but soon found another partner with whom she continues to enjoy life, love, and an intentional community they are helping to create. Sonia finds that they're not really interested in seeking out other lovers most of the time, but they value the freedom to be open to new adventures as they present themselves.

INDIA

Like China, India presents some strange paradoxes when it comes to sexuality and intimate relating. The famous erotic temple sculptures of Khajuraho and the present-day practices of existing indigenous tribal peoples in central India, the well-known writings of Kama Sutra, and the popular worship of Krishna with his thousands of wives, and legendary queens and goddesses with more than one husband all point to a culture where sexuality was celebrated and multiple partner relating was sanctioned. Waves of invaders, first the ancient Persians, then Muslims, then British, all brought their own mores to the Indian subcontinent. Uma, a psychotherapist in Mumbai (formerly known as Bombay), feels that the British are primarily responsible for the sexual repression that has prevailed in Indian society for the past century and that most Indians "have not managed to shake off yet." Prior to the arrival of the British, the upper classes and royalty were known to enjoy lovers in addition to their husbands or wives. To this day, Muslim Indians are permitted more than one wife, while the Hindu Marriage Act of 1955 prohibited polygynous marriage for non-Muslims. Nevertheless, it is still common in many villages for a man to have more than one "wife," but women's sexual freedom is usually quite restricted except, as we shall see, in some modern, urban settings.

One of the most difficult things for me about traveling in tropical India was that it is still frowned on for a woman to show bare shoulders or legs. Midriffs peeking through colorful saris, strangely enough, are perfectly acceptable as long as they are topped by short-sleeved breast coverings.

Women must cover up throughout most of Turkey and the rest of the Muslim world, where head scarves are also required in mosques, and the burka is common in most areas. In predominantly Buddhist Thailand and Cambodia, modesty is also the rule in temples or in the vicinity of the many celibate monks, but in India, this prohibition on bare skin coexists with temples filled with Shiva Lingams and sculptures depicting love making in every conceivable configuration.

Khajuraho is a popular tourist destination, and in the small town that has grown up around the temples, there are many small hotels and restaurants catering to travelers. Shiva is a strikingly handsome young Indian man who looks as though he just stepped out of one of the ancient carvings. When he learned that I was an expert on polyamory from the United States, he asked me to have dinner at his restaurant and give him some coaching. "It's easy to meet foreign women here," he told me. "Even the ten-year-old boys know that all you have to do is ask a woman if she wants to learn Tantra and you have a date." Shiva has had many love affairs with tourists who end up staying anywhere from a few weeks to a few months before moving on. "But this time it's different. It's not just a fling. Genvieve and I Skype almost every day since she went back to France. It would be easy to have other women and not tell her; lots of Indian men do that. And she could do the same, but we've talked about it, and we want to be honest with each other, to share everything. She's going to come back next year when she finishes college, but now we are apart, and we want to enjoy life but still be close to each other. The trouble is, she gets jealous when I tell her I've been with another woman. I get jealous of her too. I'm afraid she won't come next year as she's promised. It's a lot of drama! What can we do?" I gave Shiva the links to the material on my website about managing jealousy, applauded his good intentions, and gave him the cardinal rule about dealing with jealousy: never try to reason with a jealous person. Instead, breathe through the emotional upset, find support from sympathetic friends or a therapist, and talk about it when the jealousy has subsided.

Khajuraho was the spiritual capital of the Chandella dynasty, known for the flourishing of arts that took place under their long and stable reign. These exquisite temples were built over a 200-year period, beginning in the tenth century. Twenty-five of the original eighty remain, spread over a twenty-one-square-kilometer area. Because they are located in such a remote area, invaders never completely destroyed them, and like the similarly amazing ruins in faraway Ankgor Watt in Cambodia, they were covered by jungle for centuries before being discovered by westerners in the nineteenth century. It's obvious from the sculptures covering the walls of the existing temples that group sex was part of the repertoire of this accomplished culture. Scenes with every conceivable combination of sexual union abound, but they are side by side with scenes of all aspects of life, various gods and goddesses, animals, and plant life. Judging from the sculptures, despite the freedom to explore many configurations, the male/female dyad was the predominant social unit.

Perhaps this society is distantly related to the Gonds people, an indigenous tribal people still living in the forests of central India who are known for their Ghotuls. The Ghotul is thought to be a very ancient institution where young people are taught everything from crafts to ethics to farming to the arts of love. In some villages, all the young people, both girls and boys, sleep together at the Ghotul beginning in early puberty, though they still visit with their parents daily. They are given total sexual freedom and are expected to explore intimacy with everyone in the group so that they can learn who they are from the many different reflections. Pairing up is forbidden until adulthood, at which time monogamy is the rule.

The Gonds people live in modern-day Maharashtra, the same state where cosmopolitan Mumbai and Pune, site of the infamous Osho ashram, is located. Pune has become a high-tech center and is home to many Indian professionals as well as those attracted by the Ashram founded by the man first known in the West as Bhagwan Shree Rajneesh and later as Osho. Osho was well known for developing spiritual practices that encouraged people to say "yes" to the shadow—and to sexuality. He encouraged couples to break out of the confines of traditional marriage and encouraged singles to passionately follow their attractions. Jivana was one of many young Americans and Europeans who spent time at the ashram in its heyday, drawn to the chance to be in the presence of Bhagwan.

Jivana says that she felt caught in the "evolutionary wobble" while living at the ashram. All the old forms for relationship were breaking down, and there were daily therapy groups to provide a place for people to look at what was coming up for them. What Jivana discovered when she fell in love, she says, is how wounded she was. Having never experienced such love, such safety, such sublime sex, she wanted to establish a solid dyad before opening up to others, but she also wanted to honor her new partner's autonomy. Nevertheless, her partner felt this as limitation and control and they frequently argued.

Many Osho sanyasins I've known over the years have been conflicted about nonmonogamy. Osho taught that monogamy required a high level of awakeness, that it was a very high spiritual practice. He also taught that true love is not possessive, that if your beloved wishes to be with someone else, it doesn't work to try to prevent it. But without the ongoing support of the guru or at least the community, it's been difficult for many sanyasins to reconcile the two. Today, the Osho resort, as it's called, is perhaps the most Western place in all of India. Its rooms have purified air, its food is organic, the bathrooms are sparkling clean, the swimming pool is hygienic, and the large meditation hall is equipped with soundlessly closing airtight doors and frigid air-conditioning. In the required orientation meeting I attended, there were visitors from all over the world, but perhaps a third were Indian. Things have changed a lot in India in the past thirty years.

Raj Mali is a thirty-five-year-old Osho sanyasin (devotee and follower of Osho's teachings) who grew up in Pune. He is a successful corporate trainer and relationship and intimacy coach whose practice includes young polyamorous couples. Two years ago, after reading my book *Polyamory: The New Love without Limits*, Raj decided to take the leap and come out to his family. While westerners are often apprehensive about family reactions to polyamory, family is far more important to Indians. Fortunately for Raj, his family was concerned but lovingly accepting and even curious. "Initially the journey looked dangerous, but when I embraced it, it set me free. The path was laced with deep confrontation and sometimes fear, but now when I look back, it was all worth it," he says.

Raj fantasized about having an open marriage while still in high school, long before he'd ever heard of polyamory. When he shared his ideas with his friends, they ridiculed him, and his girlfriend was furious at the very idea. Realizing that for the people he knew marriage meant monogamy, or cheating, he decided not to marry. Now he's happy to be able to suggest polyamory as an option when working with couples where a secret affair is on the horizon. When I told him I was writing about polyamory in India, Raj agreed to tell me a little about one of the couples he was coaching.

Reemah and Avinash are in their late twenties and were about six months into a passionate romance when Reemah found herself struggling with jealousy for the first time in her life. When Reemah slapped Avinash on learning he was late for a meeting with her because he'd been talking with Sheela, a woman they were both friendly with, Avinish decided he'd better not have any more friendships with women but felt resentful and began to feel he needed more space from Reemah. Although he was still very much in love with Reemah, he secretly started feeling more attracted to other women. The more he withdrew, the angrier and more suspicious Reema became. As this downward spiral, which I call the "dominant woman and submissive man two-step," built, Reemah decided to seek help from Raj.

When Raj guided Reema to take her attention off of Avinash and direct it toward discovering what was underneath her jealousy, she quickly discovered that she was trying to avoid her own strong desire to experience sex with other men. Reema was caught between the judgments she'd internalized that women who slept around and didn't marry were sluts and the awareness that she wanted very much to be one of these sluts. Meanwhile, Avinash was feeling more and more torn between his attraction to his woman friend and his loyalty to Reema. He eventually allowed himself to be seduced by Sheela, and when Reema intuited this, he confessed. A major fight ensued, and they decided they should have some sessions together with Raj. He was able to help them recognize that both of them wanted to stay together and that both wanted to have sex with others but were afraid to be truthful with the other about their desires. Avinash didn't like the idea of Reema having other partners but realized that if he was going to claim this freedom for himself, it was only fair that Reema have it for herself. Faced with the prospect of breaking up or opening up, they decided together to try opening up. They are still working on managing their respective jealousies and sometimes fight about the other intimate friends in their lives, but for now they are still choosing to put each other first.

I arrived in Bombay a few weeks after the 2008 terrorist attack that left residents and tourists alike in a state of shock. Sandeep, an Indian man in his early forties who runs a small consulting firm in Bombay, was still reeling and grateful that his immediate family was unharmed. Sandeep has been married to Leela for fifteen years, and they have a six-year-old daughter. Theirs was an arranged marriage, as is still common in India; nevertheless, they came to love each other deeply. Sandeep told me that Leela is his best friend, that they tell each other everything, and that they started their business together as well. Two years ago, Leela told Sandeep that she wanted to become sexually intimate with their good friend Karna. Sandeep was very uncomfortable about this, partly because Karna was not telling his wife but also because his own jealousy was painful and intense.

He'd already downloaded my *Compersion* e-book by the time we met and had found it helpful, but he was still struggling.

Sandeep had been introduced to me online through a mutual friend, and when he heard I was coming to India, was eager to meet with me. I had coached many couples in the United States dealing with similar situations and was not surprised to find that poly hell, as some people call it, knows no national borders. I'm told it's unusual for an Indian wife to openly assert her sexual freedom and for her husband to be accepting of this, but I suspect that Sandeep and Leela are on the leading edge of a growing polyamorous movement in India. Sandeep is a thoughtful, insightful man and a professional communicator with a Western education. He is a student of Bombay advaita master Ramesh Balsekar, who teaches that it is only our thoughts about what should or shouldn't be happening that disturb the natural state of peace and happiness. Leela and Karna also have an affinity for advaita, and the threesome have attended many *satsangs* (literally translated, this means "meetings in truth") together, so I figured that they had at least some chance of working this out.

I began by acknowledging Sandeep's courage and willingness to let jealousy be his teacher and then inquired about his family of origin. As I'd guessed, Sandeep's relationship with his wife mirrored that with his mother, who was a fiery and dominating figure. His father was amiable but distant, much like Karna. Clearly, this triangle offered Sandeep an opportunity to do the inner work of healing the past, and he had the necessary skills and motivation to move through these old issues quickly, but still his marriage was at risk because Sandeep and Leela had never established a satisfying sexual relationship. I suggested that he ask Leela if she were willing to invest some time and energy in creating a sexual connection with him as well as with Karna. In India, as in the United States, it's sometimes easier for people to access their eroticism with a new partner than with the spouse they know so well.

It always seems ironic to me that, Khajuraho, Kama Sutra, and Ghotuls notwithstanding, many modern Indians have yet to undo the heavy burden of sexual repression. Yet there is evidence that this is changing. Facebook now has a "Polyamory India" group, and upper-class Indians have discovered swinging. I met Chitvan and Suresh in southern California, where they had gone to visit Sandra and Jack after meeting at a lifestyles convention in Las Vegas. Both Chitvan and Suresh are medical doctors in Delhi and have been married for fifteen years. They are an affluent, upwardly mobile, high-energy couple in their early forties who are anything but sexually repressed. Jack described his first meeting with Chitvan at one of the many lifestyles parties: "I was resting on a couch next to Sandra, and Chitvan sits down and starts fondling me. After a brief conversation with Suresh and Sandra, she grabbed me by the cock and dragged me off to the group room where she had her way with me. She was an extraordinarily skilled lover. After I came twice, I told her, 'I think I'm done.' But Suresh, who was engaged with Sandra a few feet away, heard me and said, 'Don't worry, she'll get you hard again,' and he was right, she did! I'm looking forward to visiting them in India. Chitvan has promised to throw a swing party for us there."

EUROPE

Dossie Easton, therapist and coauthor of *The Ethical Slut*, gave the keynote address at the First International Conference on Polyamory and Mononormativity held at the University of Hamburg, Germany, in 2005. Scholars from all over the world gathered to discuss the variety of ways that people in many communities structure their relationships. Organizers Robin Bauer and Marianne Pieper, who originated the term *mononormativity*, say that they wanted the conference to combine activism and academia. Dossie reports that "the German academics were concerned that I did not present a unified economic theory that addressed socialism, capitalism, class issues, and the potential for polyamory to create economic and political equality for all. They wanted to know how polyamory will help solve social problems beyond individual relationships, and I suspect they thought I was remiss in not developing such theories."[4]

Many organizers and researchers outside the United States have echoed this observation, confirming my own impression that in Europe and the United Kingdom, the polyamory movement is less focused on personal growth and more focused on the political and ecological implications of relationship choices. It also appears that the gay, lesbian, bisexual, transsexual, and queer community in Europe, the United Kingdom, and Australia are more likely to have embraced polyamory in their activism and research than their counterparts in the United States, resulting in a stronger presence abroad for polyamory within academia.

According to Robin Bauer, a gay, transsexual poly researcher, Germans use the term *polyamory* mostly to refer to committed multiple partner

relationships rather than *nonmonogamy*, which is primarily sexually motivated. Robin finds that gay men and other sexual minorities who have been
predominantly nonmonogamous in the past perceive the term *polyamory*
to apply mainly to heterosexuals and bisexuals who have not been part of
the alternative sexual community up until now and see no reason to identify with this foreign term.

The ZEGG community hasn't embraced the word *polyamory* either,
but they are a good example of the way in which many Europeans seem
more inclined than Americans to place polyamory in the context of a wider
movement for social change. They acquired a former Stasi camp in Belzig,
formerly in East Germany, outside Berlin just after the Berlin Wall came
down, that they have built into a successful community, now numbering
about sixty adults (60 percent female) and fifteen children. ZEGG is well
known for advocating nonmonogamy, although their members are free to
choose whatever lovestyle they prefer.

ZEGG founder Dieter Duhm was active in the German leftist student
movement in the 1960s, but as a young radical sociology professor in the
1970s, the mainstream left rejected him because he criticized Marxism
for its use of violent revolution. In the mid-1970s, he left academia to
explore alternative communities, including what is now the Osho ashram
in India, and set about creating his own vision of a "humanistic" community of people "with whom we can explore the interfaces of love, fear and
truth."[5] While the group began by focusing on organic agriculture, art,
ecology, and renewable energy technologies, it soon became apparent
that they would have to resolve conflicts around sexuality, jealousy, and
possessiveness. Duhm was strongly influenced by Wilheim Reich, another German socialist ostracized for his views on sex, health, and social
change. ZEGG soon became notorious for its practices of free love, and
while they received much negative coverage in the German press, they
also attracted thousands of visitors from all over the world who came to
participate in their seminars and summer camps. At ZEGG, free love is
considered an essential step toward a new culture of peace, partnership,
and sustainability. Their belief is that the only way to a free society is to
create a world where love is freed.

ZEGG first came to my attention in the early 1990s when they sent
a team of organizers to the United States. They sought the support of
the growing polyamory movement that we had established in the United
States but had a disdainful attitude toward both the spiritual and the indi-

vidualistic, apolitical brands of polyamory, which they felt predominated in the United States. Despite their socialist roots, they lost no time in competitively striving for their share of the newly booming polyamory seminar market in good capitalist fashion. In an interesting cycle of cross fertilization, their group process (called ZEGG forum) for resolving interpersonal conflicts, which incorporates elements of psychodrama, gestalt therapy, and body-centered therapies developed in the United States, caught on among a new generation of Americans who were too young to remember the encounter groups and consciousness-raising groups, not to mention the "oil parties" popular during the sexual revolution of the 1970s in the United States. ZEGG also inspired an annual two-week "Summer Camp" in the United States where the forum is taught and practiced and polyamorous people can have a brief taste of living in community with each other.

I spoke recently with ZEGG member Ina Meyer-Stoll, who, together with Achim, her partner for twelve years, now leads workshops on liberating love around the world as well as offering seminars to visitors at ZEGG. Ina is now in her late forties and has lived at ZEGG for twenty-five years. When she was a college student, she fell in love and lived with two men for a year but could not break through the personal and social conditioning against loving more than one. When a friend told her about this new community where they were teaching people how to get over their jealousy, she decided to investigate and immediately felt at home. Ina says that in her twenties and thirties, exploring sexually with different men was important to her, but then she became more interested in deep intimacy, communication, and continuity and is very satisfied with her single working partnership with Achim, although she still has a number of ongoing erotic friendships with men in the community. More recently, she has begun to feel the lack of new sexual adventures in her life and is wondering what a satisfying erotic life in the second half of life might look like.

Achim also has other lovers, and Ina admits with some embarrassment that she still experiences jealousy but that she now sees jealousy as being like having a cold, only it's her heart or her soul that's ill instead of her body. So she just slows down and takes care of herself until it passes. Knowing that her jealousy has to do with childhood wounds and feeling competitive with other women whom Achim might find sexier or more attractive doesn't make the jealousy stop, but she does find it's much easier when the other woman is someone she knows in the community, and she can go to her and talk honestly about it. Achim has suggested that they could marry so that she would feel more secure, but Ina says that she already knows he's committed to their relationship. They've tried living together with another man, but she says that one relationship is time consuming and richly nourishing enough and that she doesn't want or need more.

In the mid-1990s, Dieter Duhm and his partner Sabine Lichtenfels withdrew from ZEGG and founded Tamera, a center for humane ecology in Portugal. Perhaps because of their treatment by the media in Germany, who made them out to be a sex cult, or perhaps because they want to emphasize their underlying mission of world peace and ecological living, Tamera keeps a low profile as far as the lifestyle of its residents. However, my contacts in the polyamorous community in Portugal tell me that experiments with polyamorous relating are very much a part of the Tamera ecovillage as well.

Daniel Cardosa is a twenty-three-year-old graduate student in communication at a university in Lisbon, Portugal. Last year, he and two female colleagues presented a paper about polyamory at a European sociology conference. He describes the reaction of his colleagues to his research as "blank stares" because they don't understand it and don't take it seriously, but so far it's not hurt his career. Daniel is in a triad with his live-in girlfriend of six years, Sofia, also twenty-three, and for the past year with another woman who is a few years older. Daniel told me that "we're open to other relationships, of any kind. We usually discuss what we feel for someone else, and we tend to take things slowly so people can get comfortable with everything, giving/getting reassurance, stuff like that. So far, there's been some insecurities but nothing too gigantic that would cause a breakdown."

In early 2009, I was profiled by the Portuguese newsmagazine *Visao*, which also ran a story on Daniel and his triad and which gave a positive report on polyamory according to my Portuguese translator. Daniel says that polyamory in Portugal is probably fifteen or twenty years behind the United States as far as public awareness and acceptance goes, but he is doing his best to change that and has given many print and broadcast media interviews. While the Portuguese poly community is still small, Daniel reports that it's a "very tight and cohesive group of politically and socially motivated people" who host a blog (http://polyportugal.blogspot.com) and a website.

Daniel concurs that the political aspect of polyamory is very strong in Europe, although not all European polys are politically motivated. He feels that the crux of the issue is how to make polyamory work in a fast, ever-changing, and cosmopolitan world where, in his opinion, feminism, queer theory, and philosophy are more relevant than spirituality. Perhaps this is as much a generational factor as a cross-cultural one, but polyamorous folks in neighboring Spain feel that even though Spain (and Portugal) are predominantly Catholic countries, there is a more "live and let live" attitude toward polyamory than in the United States or the UK.

In the Netherlands, Leonie Linssen and Stephan Wik have coauthored *Love Unlimited: The Joys and Challenges of Open Relationships* (as of this writing, due out in August 2010) in both Dutch and English. Linssen is a relationship and stress management trainer and coach. At a *Loving More* conference, she explained that the book will be based on twelve case studies from her practice involving people in open relationships and "people dealing with the fact that they have feelings beyond their own partner." Earlier this year, she published her poly autobiography in Dutch, and she is a well-known advocate for polyamory awareness in the Dutch media.[6]

The Swiss have a reputation for being among the most proper and conventional people in all of Europe. But even in Switzerland, polyamory has a significant presence. Samuel Widmer is a cutting-edge psychiatrist perhaps best known as a pioneer in the authorized use of psycholytic substances in psychotherapy. He lives with two women and their ten children. Dr. Widmer is not making a cause out of polyamory, but he has written some books on it that I haven't read because they have not been translated from German. Even without personally experiencing his work, I'm sure that his expertise in the use of substances, which readily make conscious the deep conditioning and fears that prevent so many people from realizing embodied love that goes beyond the dyad, is not coincidental to his exploration of polyamory. His website states, "We are lovers. Our guru, whom we serve, is the power of love. We are no longer in competitive relationship with each other, we have envy and jealousy behind us. We have learned to rejoice in the happiness and success of others. That is why love and intimacy between us is possible, a common flowering, in which we share all the happiness and love together. Those of us who have become a vessel of love are kings and queens. Because they are the love, they are our gurus, our teachers."[7]

Dr. Widmer says that his family has attracted a lot of attention, some negative from "the normal society around us" and some from a growing community of people who are experimenting with triads and other multiple partner relationships as well as Tantric ritual. Not surprisingly, his circle includes some members of the ZEGG community in Germany, and he is also connected with several groups in India, which is how I first heard about him.

Christine is an American woman in her fifties who has lived in Switzerland for the past fifteen years. She originally moved to Switzerland with her former husband Hans and felt that they had an ideal relationship for ten years until he fell in love with a much younger American friend of theirs. Christine did her best to allow Hans the freedom to explore this relationship within the context of their marriage, but she struggled with jealousy and resentment toward the other woman, who seemed immature, irresponsible, and inconsiderate toward Christine. She was determined to take the whole situation on as a spiritual challenge and consulted me for help in managing her emotions.

While supporting her willingness to grow, I encouraged Christine to set some boundaries on what she would and wouldn't tolerate and to give herself the option of withdrawing from the marriage if her boundaries were not respected. I also recommended that she attend a seminar with Byron Katie, whose work was discussed in chapter 4. Christine took my suggestion and is now in training as a teacher of "the work." She also fell in love with a woman at the seminar and eventually decided to leave her husband and set up housekeeping with her new girlfriend Jeanette. Jeanette had identified as a lesbian all her life, but Christine had never before felt any sexual attraction toward women. All four lived together fairly harmoniously for a time, but Christine says that she is happily monogamously married with Jeanette now and has no interest in getting involved with other women—or men for that matter. Meanwhile, Jeanette has another girlfriend who has another girlfriend, and it's working out for everyone.

Since experiencing both a male and a female European partner, Christine reflects that they've provided her with a doorway into enjoying life and feeling expansive in ways that her American partners never did. "They seem to be wired differently, and simple things like taking the time to enjoy food and eating to being so playful and inventive with sex and pleasure have me completely enamored," she muses.

Komaja, based in Croatia but with representatives in many countries around the world, is another polyamorous European community. Unlike the ZEGG community, Komaja embraces bisexuality, homosexuality, and Tantric spirituality and has a clearly identified leader. While people in Komaja have a variety of lovestyles, the community feels that *zajedna*, which is their term for "group marriage," is the most desirable. Makaja, the group's founder and spiritual teacher, lives with three wives in his *zajedna* in Switzerland, and all share responsibility for parenting their four children. The group is organized into four "Tantric circles" with open marriages, group marriages, and singles making up each circle. The spiritual practices of the community, including both heart-centered singing and sexual encounters, are led by female priestesses. But while Komaja promotes sexual liberation and the art of love, it is also a very structured community with strict guidelines, including a ban on infidelity, violation of which can lead to immediate expulsion. As it says on their website, "Instead of free sex, we need free love," and, lest this be misunderstood, it then says that while love needs no restrictions, sex should always be under control. Partners are bound by "love-erotic contracts" and are expected to follow the community's sensible prescriptions for expanding sexual love without risking the well-being of partners or the security of their children.[8] I find myself put off both by guru worship and by extensive rules, but I've also noticed that strong leadership is often essential for people who are in the process of questioning their conditioning around intimacy if chaos—and dissolution—is not to prevail.

In 2003, one of Makaja's wives sent me a copy of a new English translation of his book, *Eros and Logos*, and invited me to come visit their summer school on the Croatian coast. I was curious but had other priorities at the time and so declined. However, my colleague Serena Anderlini-D'Onofrio, author of *Gaia and the New Politics of Love*, which is discussed in chapter 11, was able to spend ten days with the Komaja community in 2006.[9] She noted the slower and gentler rhythms of Europe relative to the United States and found Makaja's facilitation to be sensitive and effective. She also admired the communication skills and willingness of the Komaja members to address whatever challenges arose in the group.

After teaching all over Europe, Dossie Easton, coauthor of *Ethical Slut*,[10] reports that she was impressed by the willingness of Europeans to talk about their deep emotions. She had imagined that in Germany and England, people would be less willing to self-disclose but instead found that "they dove into talking about the emotional realties of their most painful experiences of jealousy as if they were diving into a pool in an oasis in a huge dry desert." She continues, "Europeans in my classes have been incredibly appreciative of our California human-growth-potential approach to talking about our feelings. I hear it is a new experience for many of them."

Easton also commented that access to universal health care throughout Europe and the United Kingdom supports the freedom that people have to experiment in their relationships. People in other countries can leave relationships with which they are unhappy, and they still have health care, and so do their children unlike in the United States, where leaving a marriage or a job can leave you without health insurance, she points out.

In addition, Easton found that in some cities, such as Amsterdam, women seem to feel safer and freer in expressing their sexuality than in the United States. "They had no fear that opening up about their sexuality, their fantasies, or their histories, would in any way expose them to anything intrusive or unwelcome. I was touched almost to tears by the freedom and ease with which they expressed themselves, with words and with body language. . . . In London, people were more likely to set boundaries and maintain distance to avoid potentially difficult connections."[11]

UNITED KINGDOM

Dr. Meg Barker is a thirty-five-year-old college teacher and psychotherapist based in England who is one of a handful of academic researchers, including several in the United Kingdom, to take on the unfashionable topic of polyamory. She's published a number of articles on polyamory herself and is coeditor of a new anthology called *Understanding Non-Monogamies*,[12] which is intended to bring together academic papers on polyamory, swinging, and gay open relationships from researchers in a variety of disciplines. She's also been involved with the polyamory activists in the United Kingdom who organize an annual PolyDay event in London. Dr. Barker observes that more queer activists and political people are participating in this event than in the past. In her view, "Polyamory is an interesting umbrella that includes everyone from those who want to open their relationships up sexually for very personal reasons to those who want to explore new ways of relating and change current systems for very political reasons, and everyone in between." She says that some people are questioning whether polyamory is a useful umbrella term for all those exploring "consensual nonmonogamies" or whether some people, such as swingers or gays, feel excluded or exclude themselves because they don't identify as polyamorous.

Dr. Barker says that she's "keen to keep conversations going about how people manage their relationships in these changing times." She feels it's important to demonstrate and support the diverse approaches people are taking to relating and to keep questioning the barriers and boundaries that are created and whether they serve people. Dr. Barker says that she's "drawn to ways of relating which recognize the value in various relationships rather than prioritizing sexual, romantic, or partner relationships over others." Influenced by anarchist theory as well as the Buddhist philosophy of impermanence, in recent years she's moved away from the "rigid counting of the people I was sexual with" to an awareness that all her relationships are flowing and changing and include a number of valued connections with "people and groups and places and other creatures" as well herself and the world at large.[13]

Graham Nicholls is a thirty-four-year-old artist who started his website on polyamory (http://www.polyamory.org.uk) about a year ago because he felt that the British/European perspective was a little different from what seemed relevant for Americans. This was a theme I kept hearing from Brits and Europeans, but until I chatted with Graham, I didn't have a clear idea of what was meant. He divides his time between London, where he was born; Finland, where his two bisexual female partners live; and Estonia, where he is starting a new business and two new relationships. According to Graham, Scandinavians have a greater affinity for polyamory than is the case in other European countries. He grew up in a working-class family in London and naturally gravitated toward polyamory without knowing the word or the concept. He initially heard about polyamory through websites on lesbian, gay, bisexual, transgendered, and queer issues and feminism but now emphasizes a spiritual approach. His introduction to the idea of nonmonogamy first came from reading the infamous Marquis de Sade, but he didn't like Sade's violence and negativity. After reading radical feminist Andrea Dworkin's chapter on Sade in her book on pornography, he became interested in radical feminism.

For Graham, the key issue in polyamory is not sexual morality but, rather, being open and honest in relationship. He feels that things like the pickup artist scene and the old-fashioned drunken one-night stand have sexually negative undertones but at the same time is more attracted to concepts like "relationship anarchy" than hierarchical relationships. On the basis of Internet posts and websites, he sees a greater emphasis on marriage in the United States and more interest in casual sex and general sex-positive attitudes in Europe. Graham's hope is that polyamory can be a way of raising consciousness about sexuality and relationships, not just a new form of relationship.

When Graham asked me in an instant-messaging interview what I thought about relationship anarchy, I decided I'd better get up to speed with this new term. So I contacted Andie Nordgren, a twenty-eight-year-old artist and software product manager who currently lives in London and is credited with creating and popularizing the concept of relationship anarchy in her native Sweden.[14] Andie agreed that there was little if any difference between relationship anarchy and polyamory as I defined it in my book *Polyamory: The New Love without Limits* over a decade ago: "I use polyamory to describe the whole range of lovestyles which arise from an understanding that love can not be forced to flow, or not flow, in any particular direction. Love which is allowed to expand often grows to include a number of people. But to me, polyamory has more to do with an internal attitude of letting love evolve without expectations and demands than it does with the number of partners involved."[15]

Her complaint about polyamory is that by focusing on the number of partners, it still upholds the idea that "normal" love is only between two people. In other words, even though the word *polyamory* has been substituted for *nonmonogamy*, she still sees polyamory as a variation on the monogamy/marriage paradigm. Andie, who identifies herself as a gender queer, explains, "You can compare it to the way many queers don't use the term *bisexual* even if they have relationships to both male- and female-bodied people, as the term itself indicates that there are only two genders and three sexualities (straight, bi, and gay) to choose from. The other aspect that was frustrating to me was that the polyamorous community in Sweden was still upholding a clear difference between *relationships* and *friendships*. Even if there was a lot of talk about not falling into the monogamous traps of wishing/demanding that another person be everything for you—and of course about how love was not restricted to one person—there was still a strong distinction made between those you had a relationship with and those who were just friends."

Andie says that in Sweden, the poly movement has pretty much been incorporated into the Gay Pride movement and usually operates the same way. That is, they try to claim that "we're just like you normal people, only with more partners" and try to differentiate poly from the views of it as swinging or cheating. While monogamy is still the norm for

Swedes and "mild prejudice" against polyamory still exists, most people consider it not a "super big deal" but rather a personal choice, much like in the more liberal areas of the United States. Andie found that in Sweden, polyamory was strongly linked with the bondage, discipline, dominance, submission, and sadomasochism community as well. Not surprisingly, power games are not a surefire way to warm the heart of an anarchist. For Andie, the polyamory community has "too many outdated values about gender, sexuality, power, and love and is too focused on definitions and rules and making new mental institutions for managing love relationships with several people instead of just one. Since I was interested in escaping the idea that love needed rules and institutions to survive, I never felt much at home," she says.

Andie summarizes her position as follows: "I felt a need to put another piece on the table, so that the scale of possible relationships choices didn't just go between monogamous to polyamorous but had a third, outer point   relationship anarchy. This is how I see the scale these days. Monogamy says love is only for two people; everyone knows the drill. Polyamory says love relationships can be between several people in various configurations, but there is still a difference between those who are 'partners' in various ways and those who are not. Relationship anarchy says the gray scale between love and friendship is so gray that we cannot draw a line, and thus we shouldn't institutionalize a difference between partners and nonpartners."

She realizes that from a monogamous worldview, polyamory looks no different from relationship anarchy, but to a relationship anarchist, the question "how many partners do you have?" makes no sense and is actually offensive. "The term is meant to put a useful label on an attitude that I feel is different enough from the mainstream polyamory that deals a lot with defining things like primary partners, jealousy and time management, and so on to deserve its own term," she concludes.

I'm not sure if I just happened to stumble into a bunch of anarchists in the United Kingdom coincidentally or if this emphasis on letting love flow and not making so many hierarchical distinctions between "partners," "lovers," and "friends," not to mention primaries and secondaries, is currently radiating out from Britain. In any case, this brand of polyamory is much closer to what I had in mind twenty-five years ago when I first started writing about nonmonogamy but has since been eclipsed by what radical young people are now calling "mainstream polyamory"

AUSTRALIA AND NEW ZEALAND

Australia and New Zealand, like Hawaii, and a few remaining isolated places in North America, as well as Central and South America and Asia, have more recently established dominant modern cultures existing in tandem with the original, so-called primitive indigenous people who've occupied these lands for millennia. As can be seen in the beautiful film *Ten Canoes*, the aboriginal people of Australia and New Zealand, like those of the Amazon River basin, many parts of Africa, and other remote places around the world, still have living traditions of various forms of nonmonogamy.[16] Perhaps this accounts in part for the relatively early appearance of a polyamory movement in Australia and New Zealand, largely modeled on that in the United States. While the movement is still small and struggling, it's been visible since the early 1980s and is quite well organized.

When I put out a request for information on polyamory in Australia and New Zealand, nearly a dozen leaders and organizers responded with detailed information on the histories of their local support groups in the big cities of Australia and more rural areas of New Zealand. My impression is that in Australia, poly people are still trying to find each other. The numbers are still small enough that they're quite warm and accepting of everyone. In the United States, at least in major metropolitan areas, people have long since found each other, and now they're either just living their lives outside of any identified polyamorous community or fighting about who has the one true poly way.

Anne, who runs a local polyamory group in one of Australia's bigger cities, provides a good example of the way that many Australians have been isolated from a larger community or movement and had to figure out polyamory on their own, much the way things were in the United States in the 1980s when I first started organizing. Anne says that she fell in love with her current partner over twenty years ago, when he was married with children. They were both deeply religious Christians at the time. She explains, "We didn't have a sexual affair, but the emotional connection was overwhelmingly strong. On the advice of his minister, we stopped having anything to do with each other, and I married on the rebound. If willpower could have changed how I felt for him, I would have done it. However, over the next five years, we kept running into each other, and the feelings rekindled. We tried everything in our power to manage our feelings within the context of our marriages, but the strength of our emotional connection to each other continued to outweigh our connection to our spouses. It felt like an emotional affair, even though we were as honest with our spouses as we could be.

"Eventually our marriages broke up, and we got together. However, I didn't want to be monogamous for a number of reasons. Integrity has always been extremely important to me, and I was horrified that I couldn't keep my marriage vows. I never again wanted to promise anything I couldn't guarantee I could honor. Also having been a good Christian, I hadn't really done much sexual exploration, and I wanted the freedom to do that. But my primary reason was that I never wanted to prohibit myself or my partner from something that gave us such deep joy.

"For the first five years, we struggled, largely on our own. We didn't have a word for what we were doing except 'not monogamy.' We were very cautious about who we told. We made mistakes. My partner Pete struggled with jealousy, and I was too hard on him. I had a lot of guilt left over from my Christian days. I personally had a couple of nasty experiences of utter condemnation early on, which set me back about a year in terms of confidence and willingness to explore. At first we only knew one other couple and a couple of gay friends who were nonmonogamous. We struggled with issues that our monogamous friends couldn't help us with. We felt like we had to 'make it up as we went along' to a large degree.

"At some point an academic friend who works in a related area suggested that we might be polyamorous, and we looked it up on the Internet. It was such a relief to discover that there were others like us out there, that we weren't completely weird or alone, that others considered it an ethical choice. Over time we connected with a few more nonmonogamous people, received more understanding from our close community, opened up to a few more people, and resolved more of our personal internal issues. Pete developed a life-partner relationship with Min, and we had some issues balancing our new V. However, I still struggled to find people who were really on my wavelength. I had a lot of experiences of monogamous people being frustrated with monogamy and trying out polyamory on me and then deciding it wasn't for them and shutting down from me—the scary other woman.

"I've been with Pete for sixteen years now, and he's been with Min for over ten. They live together a couple of hours away from me (it's my choice to live alone), but we stay over with each other regularly. Our triad is very stable and supportive. I have developed another life partnership, and I have some delicious lovers in my life. My poly life is as full and rich as I could ask for," Anne concludes.

For Anne and her family, finding community has been key to their happiness and well-being, and they were patient and mature enough to work through all the obstacles along the way. They trace their success in building community to the foundation created by American transplant Carl Turney in the 1980s, the rise of the Internet, and networking with other sexual "minorities," especially the bisexual and queer communities. The Australian media is getting increasingly interested in polyamory, but it hasn't really hit the headlines yet, and many Australians are still completely unaware of polyamory. Australian polys are still hesitant to talk to the media because they aren't completely "out," and they don't trust the "sensationalist infotainment programs," according to Anne. Perhaps that's why Muffy looked me up.

Muffy is a young Australian filmmaker who graduated from film school a year ago with a major in film production. Serendipity led her to make an eight-minute documentary on polyamory for her master's degree at film school after her original plan to do something on an African refugee fell through and she had to find another topic fast. "I saw an article in *New Scientist* about polyamory," she said enthusiastically, "and it got my attention." When she met the threesome who run the Sydney polyamory group, she knew she had something hot.

"This is a topic everyone has an opinion about, everyone has strong reactions to it." Muffy said that she tried to address what people are really interested in—how you make it work and how you deal with jealousy and with all the feelings that come up.

Muffy's student project was so successful that she got some development money from a major network to do a four-hour documentary series on polyamory, but it ended up not happening when the triad she was going to feature bailed out at the last minute and she couldn't find a replacement. Anne says that this is because "almost every group Muffy thought was interesting had major internal shifts or breakups or dramas." Muffy says that most of the people she's met at the support groups are just not your "average, normal-type person—lots of bisexuals, transsexuals, bigendered . . ." she trails off. Muffy wants to make a film about a very normal young family, perhaps with children, a family who is absolutely ordinary in every way—except they're polyamorous. She's hoping that she can find one in the United States, where there are so many more polys. So sorry, but it's probably hopeless, I tell her.

"Have you considered a scripted television drama with actors?" I ask her. "I'd love to be your creative consultant!" I tell Muffy that in fact I do know some families like the one she's fantasized about, but there's no way they would agree to star in her television show. I try to explain to her that even in the United States, most people who are willing to come out poly on television do so because they have nothing to lose or have something to gain, even if it's only the illusion of fame and success. But for people who already feel successful in their lives and already have "fame," even if it's only in their neighborhood or at their child's school, it just isn't very attractive to sacrifice their privacy and risk being judged or even penalized. It's very likely that any volunteers she turns up are going to be anything but ordinary. And this seems to be the case across all the cultures I've investigated.

Petula Sik Ying Ho discusses this phenomenon in her article about flamboyant young Chinese women who have leveraged their openly polyamorous lifestyle, as well as other alternative sexual practices, to create their own "charmed circles," or high-status social standing and both financial and career rewards through a politics of iconogenesis.[17] Sik describes how one women filmed herself nude and pleasuring herself while discussing an abortion and her four boyfriends. Another wrote a newspaper column disclosing the details of her polyamorous relationships—not your average Chinese girls. Options for upward mobility are fewer, and cultural restrictions on Hong Kong women are greater than in the West, so these women were taking a big risk, but they succeeded in both being effective change agents for the culture and enhancing their own life opportunities by breaking sexual and relational taboos, much like polyamorous former porn stars Annie Sprinkle and Nina Hartley have done in the United States. While many people continue to be concerned that coming out polyamorous will harm their careers, for at least some people it's been an advantage. We'll consider more weighty pros and cons for polyamory in another chapter.

10

POLYAMORY IN MYTH, ARCHETYPES, AND HUMAN EVOLUTION

Our culture places such a strong emphasis on monogamy as the only natural way for humans to relate that most people have tended to ignore evidence that suggests that people around the globe and throughout history had no such prejudice. While pair bonding is pervasive in many cultures and among many animal species, other configurations are also common. Myths and archetypes representing polyamorous unions and behaviors can be found all over the world, as can models from chemistry, physics, engineering, and even the Old Testament.

The dyad has been considered the quintessential unit for sexual reproduction, although even this is put into question by contemporary studies of animal breeding behaviors. As we discussed in chapter 1, in the animal kingdom it's sometimes the case that fertilization and optimal DNA selection are better achieved by mating with more than one partner. Meanwhile, advances in artificial reproductive technology allow single women or infertile couples to mix and match viable sperm and egg cells. As our expectations for family life shift from the bare essentials of producing offspring to fulfilling the myriad psychological and spiritual needs of highly developed human beings, the primacy of the couple is being challenged.

There *is* something very special, very romantic, about the notion of two starry-eyed lovers locked in a close embrace. There is a yearning in our hearts for union with a twin soul or soul mate. But most often, the dream of happily ever after turns out to be a fantasy that is almost the polar opposite of the reality. While most of us long for that perfect mirror, few can tolerate the reflection. As Elizabeth Gilbert puts it in her popular novel *Eat, Pray, Love*, "People think a soul mate is your perfect fit, and that's what everyone wants. But a true soul mate is a mirror, the person who shows you everything that's holding you back, the person who brings you to your own attention so you can change your life. A true soul mate is probably the most important person you'll ever meet, because they tear down your walls and smack you awake. But to live with a soul mate forever? Nah. Too painful. Soul mates, they come into your life just to reveal another layer of yourself to you, and then they leave. And thank God for it."[1]

Many people also long for a close-knit family of spiritual partners, and this experience can be too intense for most people to tolerate as well. We yearn, too, for the balance of the triangle, the eternal triangle, which does not *have* to be a blueprint for tragedy any more than the story of Romeo and Juliet has to be emblematic of the tragic fate of couples. And there is something very special about the symmetry of the square, the completeness of the four elements, the four directions, the four that is twice two. There is something special about every number, and in the natural world, combinations and subgroupings of various sizes all have their unique properties and their unique places in the overall picture.

If we insist on limiting love to two partners, we risk irreparable damage to fragile human ecosystems that thrive on diversity and complexity. Conversely, a variety of relationship niches allows everyone to find a place that fits their individual needs and desires. This kind of diversity is the hallmark of the natural world. In chemistry, elements are classified according to the number and type of bonds they will form. Imagine if the Periodic Table of the Elements was limited to hydrogen and lithium. The polyfidelitous carbon molecule would be completely out of place in an exclusively pair-bonded world.

THE TRINITY

As pervasive as the image of two opposite-gender partners is in our culture's vision of perfect love and marriage, the number 3 is mythically even more basic in a universal sense. Two is the essence of a dualistic world-

MYTH, ARCHETYPES, AND HUMAN EVOLUTION   215

view, but 3 is the number of synthesis. Three is what makes the world go around—harmoniously.

In every atom, we find the proton, or positive force; the electron, or negative force; *and the neutron, or synthesizing force.* As our knowledge of subatomic physics gets more sophisticated, it turns out there is a whole family of other particles dancing around unseen, but these three core particles determine the qualities of the atom. In music, a chord of three notes is more dynamic and powerful than one composed of only two notes. There are three primary colors, which can be combined in various ways to make all the others. In geometry, two points define a line, but three define a plane, opening up a whole new dimension.

The triangle was emphasized as the basic unit by Dr. Roberto Assagioli, founder of psychosynthesis, who combined Western psychoanalytic knowledge with the metaphysical teachings of Alice Bailey. Buckminster Fuller, the design genius who created the geodesic dome, also focused on the triangle, pointing out that it is the only self-stabilizing, constant pattern in the universe. Thus, it is the basis of all structural systems.

In Hinduism, we have the Divine Trinity of Brahma, Vishnu, and Shiva. Before the Aryan invaders brought their patriarchal trinity to India, there was Kali or Durga, the Great Mother, who contained the entire trinity within her. The trident is an ancient symbol still associated with Shiva and, in the Greco-Roman pantheon, with Poseidon or Neptune, god of the oceans and the underworld. Whether conceived of as three aspects of the one or as three different archetypal beings, the triune roles of creator, preserver, and destroyer are central to the Hindu worldview.

Perhaps the most striking example of the primacy of the triad in Western civilization can be seen in the cultural icon of the Holy Trinity—the Father, the Son and the Holy Ghost. Many have observed that the original Holy Trinity must have included not only the father and the child but also the Great Mother. The substitution of the genderless Holy Ghost for the female principle was one of many systematic changes imposed on a preexisting culture by patriarchal Judeo-Christian clergy as they molded a new mythology for our present-day society.

Another biblical triad of note is Adam, Eve, and the Serpent. Without the transformative role of the Serpent, whose challenge to patriarchal supremacy could be compared to that of Adam's first wife Lilith,[2] the history of humanity would be different indeed.

While mothers are often primary caregivers, to the extent that males take on the role of father and actively participate in rearing their offspring, even from a distance, humans experience a basic family unit of three. The infant bonds not only with the mother but also with the father. Each one of us imprints on at least two, not just one, significant others. The nature of these first nurturing relationships has great influence on all subsequent ones.

This early patterning may explain why family systems pioneers such as Dr. Murray Bowen have found that the triangle is the basic emotional molecule. Any emotional system can best be understood as a series of interlocking triangles. This is because a two-person system is inherently unstable. Where there is one bond linking two people, this sole bond must absorb any tensions between the two. When it snaps, the connection is broken. In a three-person system, there are three bonds. So the triad is potentially three times as durable. One bond can break without completely destroying the whole system, allowing time for repairs or renegotiation. If the bonds are of equal strength and flexibility, each one carries one-third of the stress, thus distributing the load and making the whole relationship more durable. This is why the triangle is the basis of structural design in engineering. In the nuclear family, a child is often pressed into service to balance the energies of the two parents. But another adult is far more appropriate for this role.

The usual portrayal of love triangles in our culture depicts strife, jealousy, and betrayal. This viewpoint is no doubt related to Greek and Roman mythology in which amoral gods and goddesses are forever cheating on their partners and hatching horrific plots for revenge. Another example of this phenomenon is Freud's interpretation of the Oedipus myth, in which the hero murders his father and marries his mother, as the basis for all manner of psychosexual disorders. According to Freud, every child secretly aims for exclusive possession of his or her opposite-gender parent and jealously strives to eliminate the competition, the third leg of the triangle, the same-gender parent.

In chapter 6, we explored more closely the influence of the parental triangle in polyamorous unions. Healthy triangles generally are based on healthy dyadic dynamics between the parents, and unfortunately this is often not the case. For now, we can simply acknowledge that dysfunctional childhood triadic programming is likely to surface and repeat itself in triadic relationships. These archetypal conflicts are deeply rooted in Western civilization and can be either transformed through conscious effort or unconsciously reenacted when the triad brings these issues to the surface.

Alongside the archetype of the neurotic or conflictual triangle, we also find examples of healing or harmonious triangles. Esoteric writings from many sources stress the balancing qualities of the third force. Without the synthesizing energies of the third, we are left alternating between two irreconcilable polarities. For example, we have the state of excitement on the one hand and depression, its opposite, on the other. The synthesis of or balance between these two is a third quality called calm or serenity. In many traditions, the archetype of the eternal triangle is associated with the feminine. The inverted triangle is a universal symbol for the yoni, or vagina. The triangle pointing upward often symbolizes the masculine, and when they are superimposed, as in the Star of David, the two triangles represent the sacred union of the masculine and feminine energies. In Hindu and Buddhist mythology, happy triads are common. Clearly, the universal archetype of the love triangle is not inherently one of jealous struggle. It is up to us to select or create a mythology to live by that heals, not hurts.

THE MÉNAGE À TROIS

The dyad may be our cultural ideal, but the ménage à trios could be our most pervasive fantasy, judging by its frequent appearance in novels, films, and visual art as well as real life. This French term has come to suggest a purely sexual liaison, but its original meaning was that of three live-in lovers. In their book *Three in Love*, Foster, Foster, and Hadady[3] tell the stories of dozens of famous and influential threesomes, from those of the eighteenth-century writer Voltaire to the nineteenth-century philosopher Friedrich Nietzsche to the twentieth-century French president Mitterrand. Their thorough research makes it clear that many of our most esteemed artists, writers, musicians, intellectuals—even politicians, royalty, and military heroes—found their sustenance and inspiration in triads.

THE SECRET DALLIANCE

One example of a healing mythology is found in the legends of the Secret Dalliance, which is the ancient Chinese term for sexual practices that extended beyond the couple. Such practices were viewed as a legitimate means of stimulating potent, even magical, powers in both men and women throughout Asia. Multiple-partner sex was also believed to rejuvenate the participants and promote longevity.

Knowledge of the sexual techniques associated with the Secret Dalliance was carefully guarded in the days of the great dynasties to enable the ruling classes to maintain their power over the common people. A man who spent himself with his first woman would be unable to satisfy the rest, so these techniques were very necessary in China, where three to twelve wives were the norm for the relatively large middle class.

In India, the Tantric Union of Three was believed to release energies more powerful and potentially more dangerous than those experienced by a couple. Texts offering special techniques for the proper channeling of these high-voltage energies warn against proceeding unless jealousy and egotism are absent.[4] Again, this knowledge was the province of adepts and nobles and was deliberately kept from the lower classes. Perhaps the sentiment that triadic relationships were not suitable for the masses partly explains why these kinds of relationships are considered so unacceptable in today's democratic West.

Surviving Taoist and Tantric texts emphasize the lovemaking of one man with two or more women, but it's likely that these reflect the imposition of a patriarchal culture on the earlier goddess-centered one, where both men and women enjoyed multiple partners. For example, dancer Muna Tseng was able to visit one of the Duhuang caves in northwestern China, Cave 465, the Secret Ancestry Cave, dating back to the eleventh century.[5] This cave, which is generally not open to the public, depicts the story of Ming Fei, a manifestation of the Taoist immortal known as Queen Mother of the West. Tseng reports that one panel shows Ming Fei holding a cup of semen saved from the height of sexual union with many men. This elixir is said to have enlightened her and given her immortality.

There is also evidence that polyandry has been practiced in the Himalayan foothills. Draupadi, the heroine of the great Indian epic the *Mahabharata*, had five husbands, all of whom were brothers. Even today, there are reports of women with more than one husband in Tibet and Sri Lanka.

Archaeological discoveries have established that even in the Middle East, where the status of women today is abysmally low, women were formerly polyamorous. Tablets dating from about 2300 B.C. that describe so-called reforms in ancient Sumer (now southern Iraq), known as the reforms of Urukagina, state that "women of former days used to take two husbands but the women of today would be stoned with stones if they did this," according to Merlin Stone in *When God Was a Woman*.[6]

TWO GENDERS OR FOUR?

Some might argue that the dyad is the primary unit because it allows the two genders to come together to make a whole. Plato, for one, wrote that in the distant past, male and female were found in a single body, but now it takes two separate individuals, and this is why we so long to find our soul mates. Rather than digressing into questioning the desirability of a belief system that teaches that we are incomplete without our "other half," let's take a look at the assumption that humans come in only two genders.

Some Native American cultures perceive that there are seven genders, not two. Likewise, twenty-first-century "gender queers" challenge the male/female dichotomy. Swedish poly activist Andie Norgren describes it this way: "My strongest alternative identity is gender queer, where I am female bodied but present in clothing, body language and appearance pretty much male, but I have no plans or desires to change my body or official sex. I'm just there in the middle, not sexualizing that or making it a big identity transition thing, just being me."[7]

One male, one female seems to be sufficient for reproduction in most cases, provided that they are genetically compatible but not overly similar genetically,[8] but in terms of completion, several astute observers have noticed that 4, not 2, is the magic number. The quadrinity is the archetypal number of completion in the natural world. We have four directions: north, south, east, and west; four elements: earth, air, water, and fire; and four seasons: winter, spring, summer, and fall, just to name a few examples.

Spiritual teacher Leslie Temple Thurston has put forth an elegant tool for transcending polarities of any kind that relies on the square.[9] When thinking about any polarity, we can always look at it from two perspectives: that which we desire and that which we fear. So the basic polarity, *polyamory* and *monogamy*, for example, can be conceptualized as occupying four quadrants: desire for polyamory, fear of polyamory, desire for monogamy, and fear of monogamy. Usually, at least one of these quadrants is unconscious. When we become aware of the feelings and motivations associated with the blank square, the graceful resolution of completion often occurs as if by magic.

When it comes to gender, a similar quadratic equation exists. Gina Haddon[10] brilliantly describes the existence of active and receptive expressions for both masculine and feminine that she links to the functions of different sexual organs. She argues that *active* and *receptive* are the basic polarity and that these are *not* gender linked. Our culture tends to recognize only the active masculine, or phallic masculine, as symbolized by the erect penis. We overlook the receptive masculine, or testicular masculine, whose qualities include protection and constancy, even though the testicles are far more enduring than a fleeting erection. In studies of mythology, these are sometimes referred to as the solar masculine, represented by gods such as Apollo, and the lunar masculine, represented by Poseidon, god of the oceans and the underworld.

Conversely, our culture has exclusively identified the feminine with the receptive as exemplified by Mary, Mother of Jesus. This gentle, nurturing aspect of the feminine is linked with the breasts. But the feminine also has its active expression as evidenced by the birthing womb. Anyone with direct experience of childbirth knows that this quintessential aspect of the feminine is anything but soft and yielding. Fierce goddesses such as Kali and Durga in India or Pele in Hawaii are known for their sometimes violent anger. In Western civilization, we have Joan of Arc and Deborah, the female warrior and judge in the Old Testament. Mary Magdalene, who many now believe to be the consort of Jesus and mother of his child, has been presented in the New Testament as a prostitute rather than a priestess of the reigning active female deity.

With the active feminine and receptive masculine genders written out of our foundational myths, the four genders are reduced to two. Of course, just as both women and men have masculine and feminine qualities, we all have both active and receptive qualities. Nevertheless, in most people, one type predominates, and in the dyad, only two of these types are present. Is it any wonder that couples often have a sense of something missing?

POLYAMOROUS ARCHETYPES

Polytheistic cultures around the world, including Native American, African, and Celtic cultures, have also honored the power of sexualove and lack the

Christian bias toward monogamy. It is beyond the scope of this book to explore all these traditions, but brief mention of a few specifics will suggest the dramatically different perspective on monogamy found in other cultures.

Native American teacher Harley Swiftdeer describes the talent for sexualove as a special gift, similar to a gift for music or for athletic ability. Such a gift may be chosen as a person's *giveaway*, or contribution to society. This lover archetype is very different from our culture's image of the driven nymphomaniac or the irresponsible Dionysian lady's man. Furthermore, the Native American archetype of the healer encompasses the use of an abundant erotic energy for healing. A similar archetype is known in Tibetan mythology as Sky Walking Woman. She is the free spirit who will not be possessed by any individual but whose life energy has the power to revitalize those who become intimate with her.

In the West, one of the most pervasive polyamorous archetypes is Aphrodite, Greek goddess of love and beauty. To the Romans, she was Venus. In earlier times, she was known as Inanna, Astarte, Ishtar, or Isis. The Hindus call her Parvati, and she is sometimes described as the wife of Shiva. She is the feminine essence before being divided into madonna and whore.

Jungian analyst Jean Shinoda Bolen[11] calls Aphrodite the *alchemical goddess* because she alone among the Greek gods and goddesses had transformational power. She was also unique in that, while she had more lovers than any other goddess in Greek myth, she was not victimized and never suffered from her numerous love affairs as did most of the other goddesses. Neither was she jealous or possessive. Unlike her counterparts, she was allowed freely to choose both her husband and her many lovers. Aphrodite inspired poetry, communication, and creativity as well as love. She is still renowned for her powerful magnetism. Some modern women who've embodied this archetype are Isadora Duncan, the inventor of modern dance; Emma Goldman, the early feminist anarchist and free love advocate; and the pop music star Madonna.

Aphrodite's liaison with Hermes, god of communication (called Mercury by the Romans), produced the bisexual, androgynous Hermaphroditus. Her long-term union with Ares, god of war (Mars to the Romans), produced a daughter, Harmonia. Thus, love and war combined to give rise to harmony. The six-lobed Flower of Aphrodite is an ancient symbol found all over the world. It symbolizes the power of this archetype to generate growth and produce new life, and there is nothing remotely dyadic about it.

Classical Greek civilization is often cited as the primary root of today's Western cultures. Interestingly enough, neither monogamy nor romantic pair bonding was emphasized in Greek mythology or in everyday life in ancient Greece. While customs varied among the different city-states, marriages were arranged for financial and political reasons, and love was not part of the equation.[12] Unlike the contemporary arranged marriages still common in India, for example, where attention is given to the likelihood of compatibility between the betrothed and where it is hoped that love will develop over time, love between husband and wife was not even considered desirable in classical Greece. The wife's role was to provide heirs for her husband and manage his household while he enjoyed affection, sex, and companionship with a variety of women courtesans and hetaerae and perhaps men and boys as well.

In India, among the Gonds people, who are an indigenous tribe still living in the forests of modern-day Maharashtra in central India, young people live together in a coed youth house where boys and girls are given total sexual freedom and encouraged to experience intimacy with everyone in the group. Pairing up is forbidden until adulthood, at which time monogamy is the rule. This custom is thought to be very ancient. Verrier Elwin, an anthropologist who lived among these people for many years and eventually married into the tribe, once said that their message is "that youth must be served, that freedom and happiness are more to be treasured than any material gain, that friendliness and sympathy, hospitality and unity are of the first importance, and above all that human love—and its physical expression—is beautiful, clean and precious, is typically Indian."[13]

In Hawaii prior to the arrival of westerners, the ancient 'ohana, or extended family, was—and still is—central to the lives of Hawaiians. Prior to the influence of Christian missionaries and, before this, settlers from Tahiti, the Hawaiian culture was one in which men and women were equals. Both genders sometimes took more than one mate, and all shared responsibility for the children regardless of biological parentage. This custom was common among both royalty and commoners. If partners separated, all remained part of the same 'ohana. In the Hawaiian language, the same word, *punalua*, applies to multiple spouses, the unrelated spouses of siblings or cousins, or to former and current mates. *Punalua* were recognized and treated as family, and while jealousy sometimes arose, it was not frequent, perhaps because it was considered disgraceful and contrary to the spirit of *aloha*, which is roughly translated as "love."[14]

AN EVOLUTIONARY PERSPECTIVE

Speculation about the mating habits of prehistoric humans as well as observation of present-day nonhuman primates are other sources of data often called on to validate our current conjugal practices. It's interesting to note that most scholars don't bother to ask whether males prefer or will accept multiple mates. It's assumed that the male will gladly take on as many females as he can gain access to. The big question is always whether females will accept more than one male or, sometimes, whether her consorts are willing to share her with other males.

As we discussed in chapter 1, despite the unscientific but well-publicized explanatory fictions invented by some culture-bound twentieth-century sociobiologists that treat monogamy as an evolutionary mandate, the weight of evidence suggests that early humans were not monogamous.

Prominent evolutionary biologist Lynn Margulis[15] points out that the erect penis of the human male is about five times larger than that of a gorilla. Human testicles are also much larger than those of gorillas and orangutans. Among the great apes, only the wildly promiscuous chimpanzees have bigger testicles than humans. Why is this? Probably it is an evolutionary adaptation to *sperm competition*, which exists if two or more males copulate with the same female within a period of days. The one with the largest, best-timed, and deepest penetrating ejaculation will be most likely to impregnate her. Consequently, the genes for large penises and testicles are more likely to be passed on.

This theory is supported by the discovery that in species of monkeys and apes with the highest ratios of testes to body weight, the females often mate with many males. For example, with chimpanzees, a species that has one of the highest ratios, the troop is usually composed of genetically related males that hunt together and that are willing to sexually share rather than exclusively possess a female. And female chimps in heat are inclined to encourage as many males to have a go as they can round up. This could be viewed as a precursor for early forms of *group marriage*, in which a group of related males bonded with a group of related females.

Further evidence cited by Margulis for the existence of sperm competition in humans is the discovery that men who know or suspect that their mate has not been monogamous actually produce more sperm and more semen than those who believe that their wives have no other lovers. Jealousy, she concludes, is an aphrodisiac.

But jealousy can also function to motivate other behaviors, termed *sperm competition avoidance.* The huge gorilla with his one-inch-long erection and tiny testicles doesn't need a big penis to gain an evolutionary advantage. The alpha male simply prevents others from gaining access to the fertile females in his "harem." This pattern is more common in species where the male is significantly larger and more powerful than the female, a possible precursor to the form of polygamy practiced by biblical patriarchs and by patriarchs throughout the Arab world today.

Orangutans, which also have relatively tiny penises, are more likely to practice something called *takeover avoidance.* That is, the mated pair remain alone and isolated in the jungle. Sperm competition is not an issue because there are no other contenders. One might see this idiosyncratic development, without pushing the extremes too far, as a possible precursor for our honeymoon custom and the exclusivity of the nuclear family.

Anthropologist Robert Smith[16] speculates that monogamous (takeover avoidant or sperm competition avoidant) *Homo sapiens* may have been better fighters than their promiscuous well-hung (sperm-competing) *Homo erectus* predecessors. Consequently, cooperative *Homo erectus* males, failing to protect their females from control by jealous and violent *Homo sapiens*, gradually disappeared.

Another perspective on evolutionary precedents for nonmonogamous behavior can be found in the observations of anthropologist Sarah Blaffer Hrdy.[17] She points out that in primate species where the female mates with many different males, all the males in the troop are likely to be protective of her and her offspring. But in harem-type troops, males will kill nursing infants sired by another male. Thus, we could speculate that men and women have different evolutionary agendas. The female's goal is to ensure the survival of all her offspring by enlisting the support of as many males as possible. The male's goal is to protect only those offspring that he knows to carry his genes and to eliminate all others. We might call this *postnatal sperm competition avoidance.* This could be viewed as a possible precursor to genocide.

THE BONOBO WAY

Perhaps the strongest evidence of a biological basis for polyamory comes from observations of the bonobo chimpanzee. Bonobos, also known as pygmy chimpanzees, are found only in a small area of Zaire in central Africa. Nothing was known about their behavior in the wild prior to the 1970s. At first, they were thought to be juvenile common chimpanzees, but it turns out that they are a distinct species. Bonobos, unlike other chimps, frequently copulate face-to-face, and the females are sexually receptive throughout their ovulation cycle.[18] Observers agree that bonobos have a propensity for sharing sexual pleasure with a variety of partners independently of reproductive purposes. In fact, genital play is used extensively both across and within genders as a means of bonding within the group and defusing potential conflicts.

Male bonobos may use sex to reconcile with each other after an aggressive encounter, and females use sex to reinforce social ties or relieve tension. Bonobo females also build powerful alliances with each other through sexual sharing, a strategy that is thought to explain the peaceful and egalitarian relations between bonobo males and females. Unlike other primate species, such as common chimpanzees or baboons, bonobo females aren't afraid of males and live in mixed-gender groups. Although the males are physically larger and stronger, they don't dominate the females sexually or in any other way.

This discussion of primate mating patterns should not be interpreted as support for the notion that human sexuality is *merely* an extension of our genetically determined animal natures. However, it should be apparent from this brief discussion that the argument that monogamy is the only natural form of bonding has little basis in the study of primate sexual behavior—quite the contrary, as humans are genetically closer to bonobos than any other species and bonobos are happily polyamorous. They are also on the verge of extinction, but this does not appear to be a result of their mating patterns. In fact, we could speculate that it is their mating patterns that have allowed them to survive this long.

POLYAMORY AND THE PRE/POST FALLACY

Transpersonal psychologist Ken Wilber[19] draws our attention to an error that many of us make when looking at the evolution of human consciousness. He observes that we confuse the undifferentiated consciousness typical of primitive peoples, young children, and psychotics with the transcendental unitive consciousness of the mystic or saint. In other words, we mistakenly equate the undeveloped state with the highly developed state that it superficially resembles.

This same error is prone to occur when we look at the mating behaviors and family structures of primates and early humans. Evolution tends to follow a spiral, repeating a cyclic pattern that constantly brings us back to the same place but at a higher level. Consequently, group marriages in prehistoric times may resemble the group marriages of the twenty-first century in that they include the same number of partners. But the dynamics of the relationships are likely to be very different. Similarly, the image of polygamy as male-dominated harems of females has little in common with the voluntary multiple-partner relationships that men and women choose today. Neither does forced monogamy directly correspond with a conscious choice of limiting oneself to one life partner.

Polyamory is not a throwback to more primitive modes of sexual relating. Neither is cosmic consciousness a kind of schizophrenic regression. Instead, polyamory may be a more complex form of relationship for men and women who have already mastered the basics of intimacy and are prepared to evolve into more complex social organisms. By the same token, to regard polyamory as the end point of evolution would be the height of arrogance. No doubt, the evolutionary spiral has many more turns yet to come.

Science-fiction writers Spider Robinson and Jeanne Robinson explore the idea of polyamory as a contributing factor to an evolutionary leap in human consciousness in their novel *Stardance*.[20] The story revolves around the founding of the first zero-gravity, off-planet dance troupe and the subsequent use of dance to communicate with extraterrestrials. The requirements of weightless dancing soon led the group into a transparently intimate and synergistic group marriage that appears to be the ultimate manifestation of renowned futurist Teilhard de Chardin's prophetic observation that "we see Nature combining molecules and cells in the living body to construct separate individuals, and the same Nature, stubbornly pursuing the same course but on a higher level, combining individuals in social organisms to obtain a higher order of psychic results."[21]

THE FUTURE OF LOVE

Biologists find that some species respond to environmental threats to their survival by gathering into highly interdependent groupings. A bonded group is able to thrive under conditions, such as those found in outer space, that would be fatal to isolated individuals or mating pairs. Using group synergy, a bonded group can increase the efficiency with which the basic functions, such as the input and distribution of nutrients and the co-ordination of activities, are performed. In the case of humans, functional multiadult families have the capacity to share essential items, such as food, shelter, and information, while assisting in the creation of valuable products and services. The family's reproductive and child-rearing capacity can also be enhanced; this has been a major consideration for centuries by those advocating patriarchal-style polyamory.

Philosopher Dane Rudhyar was among the first twentieth-century writers to emphasize the transformational role of polyamorous relationships in human evolution. Rudhyar acknowledges that the deep love and bonding required for a group to effect core changes among individuals can occur in the presence of an authentic guru or spiritual teacher as well as in closed monastic contexts. Without these supports, he asserts that sexualove, which is "polyvalent" but still focused within a small group, can also serve a transformational purpose. Writing in the earliest days of the twentieth-century sexual revolution, Rudhyar saw it this way: "What is needed now . . . is a new type of group relationship in which the individual ego-patterns, and the conjugal tensions can be absorbed, smoothed out and harmonized by a sense of common dedication to a vital social-cultural and spiritual purpose—a transforming purpose. What is needed is a group of a few adults, perhaps from four to ten, which can provide a varied and loving, but not possessive and complex-ridden environment in which children may grow up in multiple interplay. . . . The seed group should not be con-ceived in terms of 'hedonistic' purpose—i.e., for the sake of pleasure and comfort—but rather in terms of what I would call a heroic determination to help create a new type of social consciousness based on an open, unpos-sessive and polyvalent love."[22]

Whether humans as a whole are ready to make the evolutionary leap to love beyond the couple is another question, as we have seen in previous chapters.

11

THE COSTS AND BENEFITS
OF POLYAMORY

While polyamorists have often been accused of being irresponsible and selfish hedonists, the reality is that the potential benefits of practicing polyamory extend far beyond the personal to encompass transformative impacts on our whole culture. The difficulties associated with polyamory affect primarily the individuals directly involved. Despite the fears of fundamentalist religious groups that have concerns about morality and family values, when polyamorous relationships succeed, they strengthen families and instill a greater sense of responsibility and integrity in those concerned. These gains have often exacted a cost from the pioneers who sacrifice their sense of personal control, their familiar conditioning, and perhaps the acceptance of family and social institutions when they challenge the status quo. When polyamorous relationships fail, those caught up in them pay the same price as those in successful relationships but without reaping the same rewards.

I admit I have a bias. Based on my understanding of the critical challenges facing humanity at the dawn of the twenty-first-century, which include environmental pollution, global warming, impending shortages of fossil fuels, clean drinking water, nontoxic food, overpopulation, economic crises, and the threat of war, epidemics, and natural disasters, I have a hard time seeing how polyamory could make any of these difficulties any worse. Quite the contrary, there are many reasons to think it might help.

Any kind of successful loving relationship is a boon to those directly involved in it. The main difficulty with polyamory is that it's hard to do it well. In fact, for some people, it's probably impossible, but the same could be said for monogamy. In a recent interview, psychiatrist Judith Lipton, coauthor of *The Myth of Monogamy*, commented, "It's realistic that some people can mate for life in the same sense that some people can play the Beethoven violin concerto or other people can ice-skate beautifully or learn a new language."[1]

The social and ecological problems associated with monogamy are problems not so much with monogamy per se as with a grudgingly tolerated monogamous union embedded in the nuclear family and precariously held in place by religious and civil institutions. The nuclear family is a relatively recent social experiment and is quickly becoming a relic of the past. Numerous critics from many disciplines have thoroughly exposed the dysfunctions of the nuclear family, but no one is talking about what will take its place. It would benefit us all to encourage experiments with other possibilities, and polyamory is certainly one candidate.

Lest we rush blindly into this exploration, let's begin by taking a brief look at some of the problems associated with polyamory. Most people have been overexposed to criticisms of polyamory. Unfavorable comparisons with monogamy are still the norm in our culture even when accusations of immorality are withheld. Consequently, the downside of polyamory requires less elaboration than its benefits, but this should not be seen as a dismissal of the very real liabilities associated with polyamory. After a mention of these, we'll take a look at how polyamory can make a contribution to the planet as a whole before considering its personal and social benefits.

THE PRICE OF POLYAMORY

While polyamory offers many advantages over enforced monogamy,* polyamory presents numerous problems of its own. Some of these, such as social disapproval and discrimination, are artifacts of old structures and institutions that may well diminish in coming years. Others, such as a dearth

---

*Recall that the definition of polyamory given in chapter 1 includes freely chosen monogamy, which does not involve an ironclad agreement to maintain sexual exclusivity in the diversity of forms that make up polyamory.

of positive role models and perhaps even the prevalence of jealousy, are also likely to be temporary. But other difficulties with polyamory, such as the time demands and the emotional complexity of interacting intimately with more people, appear to be inherent to this lovestyle. Let's consider each of these potential costs and detrimental impacts in turn.

For many people, the risk of rejection by family, neighbors, friends, and coworkers leads them to reject polyamory. For those who are strongly motivated to be seen in a positive light by others, this consideration alone is a deal breaker. I was once married to a man whose personality was a near-perfect fit for polyamory. He had no particular desire for sexual exclusivity, he had strong interpersonal skills, and he was generally adventurous, but because being respected and admired in his community was of primary importance to him, polyamory was not at all attractive to him. Polyamory was very attractive to Jonathan, a man with similarly appropriate personality traits who consulted me about his concern that if he were inadvertently "outed," it would reflect badly on his wife, Victoria, who was beginning a new career as a pastor. Jonathan and Victoria had successfully opened their marriage over a decade ago, and now he was conflicted about her request that he return to monogamy. I had to advise him that their fears were realistic: monogamy would be a far safer choice at this juncture in their lives.

Social sanctions serve to keep couples such as Jonathan and Victoria, who would be potentially excellent role models, safely out of sight. I know of several group marriages and open marriages whose highly functional partners have chosen to keep their intimate lives private because they did not want to jeopardize other important work they were doing in the world by exposing themselves to criticism of their preferred lovestyle. Politics is one field in which polyamory presents an ever-present danger, particularly in an era where strategists desperate to win an election will publicize personal information that was once off limits to journalists. For example, former presidential candidate John Edwards was forced to withdraw from his campaign for the Democratic nomination in 2008 after his extramarital affair made headlines, as was front-runner Senator Gary Hart in 1987. President Bill Clinton was impeached by the House of Representatives but acquitted by the Senate in 1998. In European countries, nonmonogamy is less of a political liability, but the prudent politician is still unlikely to announce that he or she is a supporter of polyamory. With so many politicians being exposed as nonmonogamous, those whose extramarital activities are consensual are easily lumped together with those who are cheating. Some have speculated that it might even be less politically damaging to apologetically admit an affair than to come out as polyamorous.

Nonmonogamous relationships have a reputation for creating emotional chaos and drama that is only partly a result of broken agreements and dishonesty, which are no more characteristic of polyamory than of monogamy. As we discussed in chapter 4, if partners are able to relate with self-responsibility and integrity, drama need not be part of polyamorous relating. But as long as our culture endorses monogamy and socializes our young people to expect sexual exclusivity, we can expect jealousy to be a major obstacle. While polyamory has the potential to reduce stress, it also has the potential to increase stress. When a stressful moment in a polyamorous relationship coincides with other stressors, an emotional meltdown may result and is often attributed to polyamory even though the relationship issues are only one factor.

Emotional upheaval, on the other hand, may well go with the territory, at least until our brains have been rewired. Even when people think they have grown beyond jealousy and fear of abandonment, they can be surprised by a new situation that reactivates old issues. Some might see this as a wonderful opportunity to clear up emotional baggage they didn't know they had, but others would prefer to avoid these painful reminders. For example, Cheryl was relieved to have found a sense of peace and stability in her triadic relationship with Paul and Leslie after the year of emotional ups and downs that ensued when Leslie told Cheryl she wanted a sexual relationship with their friend Paul. When Paul asked if his former partner Harry could join them for dinner, Cheryl found herself enraged for reasons she couldn't understand but soon realized she was afraid this dinner might be the start of another roller-coaster ride. She wasn't sure if she was more afraid that Paul might leave her and Leslie to go back to Harry or that Harry might end up expanding their threesome to a foursome. She liked her life just as it was and didn't want any more changes. Living in the moment was a challenge for Cheryl, who found it hard to trust that change might make a good thing even better.

Challenges with time management and coordination are probably an inevitable part of polyamorous relating. As one member of an eight-person intimate network put it, "Have you ever tried to get eight people to agree on where to go for dinner and then get them all out the door at the same time?" This kind of dilemma is common but, while relatively trivial, can take its toll over time. Nevertheless, it is likely to be less emotionally loaded than a conflict over who is going to sleep with whom when everyone's preferences are different and time options are scarce.

Sally was leaving town the next day on an extended business trip. Oscar and Frank each wanted her to spend her last night alone with them. "I honestly didn't have any preference," Sally moaned, "and maybe that was the problem because they both wanted me to decide, and I didn't want to. I would have been happy for all of us to stay together, but that wasn't what they wanted. We ended up spending most of the night talking about what to do and why." Even when decisions about how much time to spend with different partners are not an issue, simply fitting several relationships into a busy life can send some people racing back to monogamy.

With all these difficulties, is polyamory worth the struggle? Why would anyone want to swim upstream when they don't have to?

POLYAMORY AND THE GAIA HYPOTHESIS

Feminist humanities professor Serena Anderlini-D'Onofrio has woven together fact and theory from widely disparate fields to present a case for the value of polyamory and other nonnormative sexualoving expressions to preserve human life on planet Earth. She views polyamory as a school for love that teaches a way of feeling and thinking that is crucial for our survival as we enter the twenty-first-century.

One of the central themes of her *Gaia and the New Politics of Love*[2] is the utility of the hypothesis originally put forth in scientific terms by James Lovelock[3] and Lynn Margulis and widely adopted by ecofeminist philosophers, neopagans and others that planet Earth, or Gaia, is not mere inert matter but has a consciousness like an animated, self-regulating organism. This point of view has been pervasive among indigenous people the world over for millennia and is the basis for all nature-based spirituality. Anderlini-D'Onofrio traces the development of modern religious and scientific thought that views Earth as an inert object. This worldview happens to correlate both with the rise of monogamous marriage as the only legitimate sexual expression and, as many observers have noted, with the increasingly life-threatening destruction of our environment.

The value of accepting the Gaia hypothesis, she asserts, is that it moves us away from a course of irreversible environmental destruction and human suffering and toward greater justice and ecosocial sustainability. In

her words, "Hypothesizing Gaia in our era is like hypothesizing helio-
centrism in Galileo's. It helps the world shed needless fears from current
dogmas, like the idea that love is a crime or a disease, or that we need to
fight preventative wars against terrifying enemies, and it gets us to look
reality in the face."[4]

Another major theme for Anderlini-D'Onofrio is the concept of symbiotic reason. She defines symbiosis as a way of sharing bodies in which
both host and guest benefit. In biology, this refers to phenomena such as
beneficial bacteria found in the digestive tract of many species. We might
also apply the term to the presence of humans and other species living in
the body of Gaia. Symbiosis classically describes the relationship between
a pregnant woman and her fetus. In Freudian psychoanalytic thought, the
term *symbiotic* refers to a pathologically dependent maternal relationship
carried beyond the appropriate developmental stage. Instead, Anderlini-
D'Onofrio argues for a new understanding of symbiosis as "the wellspring
of a mode of reasoning that appreciates the sharing of bodies as resources
for fun and pleasure and does not diagnose it as unhealthy or perverse."[5]
Not only is symbiotic reason crucial to sustainability, she says, but it's also
closely related to the practice of polyamorous love.

Patriarchal values have placed independence and logic above symbiosis
or *inter*dependence and direct bodily awareness—with disastrous results.
Rational science has been revealed as lacking the objectivity on which its
alleged superiority is based. Symbiotic reason, which leads us to think in
terms of the whole rather than isolated parts, is the cure, according to
Anderlini-D'Onofrio and countless other contemporary thinkers. As she
expresses it, "I believe that the political problem of today is a problem of
love because only hatred and fear can cause people to construct enemies
that do not exist while they ignore the most serious and impending issues.
I propose holism as an ecologically sound approach to biopolitical issues
that heals the thought system that causes anxiety, rather than attacking the
enemies this system constructs. Love is therefore the problem that is also
the solution of modernity's diseases and the absurd position these diseases
put us humans in. In homeopathic terms, love is the disease that is the
cure. Indeed, if as humans aware of being mere cells in Gaia's organism
we could love as selflessly as the two unicellular organisms who die to
merge into one larger symbiotic being, we could perhaps cure ourselves of
modernity's diseases."[6]

Anderlini-D'Onofrio takes this line of thought a step further by emphasizing the mutual sharing of oxytocin-mediated bonding in symbiotic styles of love, which, by her definition, include polyamory. Oxytocin is a hormone well known for its role in bonding a breast-feeding mother to her newborn infant. More recently, the action of oxytocin in promoting bonding of sexual partners, at least temporarily, has been highlighted. Oxytocin produces feelings of calm, love, and connection. Could it be the antidote to the anxieties of modern life still driven by the adrenaline-driven fight-or-flight syndrome? At the risk of oversimplifying, this could be likened to the famous slogan of the 1960s peace movement, "Make love, not war," in terms of neurotransmitters.

Polyamorous people, Anderlini-D'Onofrio asserts, have developed practices that allow the establishment of gradual levels of intimacy, including playful touch, cuddling, snuggling, spooning, and inclusive sexual play. "Because of their heavy reliance on touch, connectedness, nonviolence, and a subtle knowledge and practice of intimacy, the styles of love invented by bi and poly people promote the activation of the hormonal cycle of oxytocin."[7] Of course, these practices are not limited to the polyamorous, but they are often avoided, particularly in group settings, by those who are fearful of temptations to stray from their monogamous vows.

THE NEUROBIOLOGY OF PLEASURE AND VIOLENCE

Dr. James Prescott is a developmental neuropsychologist and former researcher at the National Institute of Child Health. On the basis of extensive laboratory research with animals, he theorized that the deprivation of physical sensory pleasure is the principal root cause of violence. His experiments showed that in animals, pleasure and violence have a reciprocal relationship. The presence of one inhibits the other. In other words, when the brain's pleasure circuits are "on," the violence circuits are "off" and vice versa. A raging, violent animal will abruptly calm down when electrodes stimulate the pleasure centers of its brain. Stimulating the violence centers in the brain can terminate the animal's sensual pleasure and peaceful behavior.[8]

Do these animal studies apply to humans? Prescott maintains that a pleasure-prone personality rarely displays violence or aggressive behaviors and that a violent personality has little ability to tolerate, experience, or enjoy sensuously pleasing activities. As either violence or pleasure goes up, the other goes down in humans as well as animals. Prescott found further evidence for his theory by examining data correlating extramarital sex taboos with sexism, crime, and violence in cultures around the world. According to Prescott, "The data clearly indicates that punitive-repressive attitudes toward extramarital sex are linked with physical violence, personal crime, and the practice of slavery. Societies which value monogamy emphasize military glory and worship aggressive gods."[9]

Deep-ecology advocate Dolores LaChapelle was one of the first twentieth-century writers to discuss sex and intimate relationships in an ecological context. She views the breakdowns in so many modern relationships as a direct result of placing too much emphasis on the romance between two people and losing sight of the larger whole in which we are all embedded. In her encyclopedic *Sacred Land, Sacred Sex,*[10] she draws on indigenous wisdom the world over to paint a vivid picture of the ways in which multipartner sex has traditionally served to bond the group, diffuse potential conflict, and strengthen the connection to the land. She cites many examples of both ancient and modern native peoples whose customs and rituals incorporate sex as "natural, inevitable, and sacred because it's part of the whole inter-relationship of humans and nature in that place."[11]

One account is from a woman anthropologist who was traveling through the jungle with a woman friend from the tribe and the woman's husband. When they stopped to camp for the night, her friend was making love with her husband and asked if she wanted to join in. She describes the experience as natural, playful, tender, and bonding for the two women.

In many of these cultures, as in the lovestyle now called polyamory, pair bonding is one option among many, and couples expect to include others in their intimacy or relax their boundaries when the situation arises. Couples as well as other grouping and singles all participate in seasonal festivals involving ritual sex to "increase the energy not only between man and woman but within the group as a whole and between the humans and their land."[12]

Prescott's previously mentioned research revealed that cultures like these are significantly less violent than those that disallow extramarital sex. While modern Western thinking generally regards fertility rites as merely superstitious, if not immoral, LaChapelle, like Anderlini-D'Onofrio and Prescott, describes a biological basis for their positive effects.

LaChapelle explains it this way: "In ritualized sex, which is not confined to the genital area, the entire body and the brain receive repetitive stimuli over a considerable period of time. This leads to 'central nervous system tuning.' To briefly summarize, if either the parasympathetic nervous system or the sympathetic nervous system is stimulated, the other system is inhibited. Tuning occurs . . . when there is such strong, prolonged activation of one system that it becomes supersaturated and spills over into the other system so that it, in turn, becomes activated. If stimulated long enough the next stage of tuning is reached where the simultaneous strong discharge of both autonomic systems creates a state of stimulation of the median forebrain bundle, generating not only pleasurable sensations but . . . *a sense of union or oneness with all*. This stage of tuning permits right hemisphere dominance; thus solving problems deemed insoluble by the rational hemisphere. Furthermore, the strong rhythm of repetitive action as done in sexual rituals produces positive limbic discharge, resulting in increased social cohesion; thus contributing to the success of such rituals as bonding mechanisms."[13]

Of course, polyamory does not necessarily involve such exotic activities, but as a philosophy of love, it provides a context in which erotic ritual is possible without prohibitions based on a belief in entitlement to sexual exclusivity as proof of commitment or fidelity. What polyamory does require is a more altruistic, unconditional type of love than is common in monogamous unions and that naturally arises from a felt sense of oneness. While monogamy, of course, also thrives on unselfish love, it can survive more easily than polyamory in its absence.

POLYAMORY AS A TRAINING GROUND FOR UNCONDITIONAL LOVE

In my book *The Seven Natural Laws of Love*,[14] I discuss the universal principles that govern the flow of love in the world, just as the laws of physics govern the interactions of matter and energy. Most people are aware that as our understanding of the physical nature of reality has grown, physics has undergone several paradigm shifts. The physics that is taught in universities today is not the same physics that was taught in the nineteenth or even the twentieth century. A paradigm shift is also taking place in our comprehension of love, but there are few resources available for integrating this new understanding. Polyamorous relationships are one of these precious resources. While any intimate relationship is a training ground for love, polyamory inevitably brings several "laws" of love front and center, where they cannot fail to get our attention.

One of these principles is what I've referred to as the *law of consciousness*. In the old paradigm for love, we think of love of as a substance, something that can be given or received, as something that can be lost or taken away. We imagine that love is like a pie that can be cut into slices. The bigger your piece, the less there is for me. In the new paradigm, we recognize that love is not an object. Rather, love is an energy, a vibration, a state of consciousness. The image is that of a radio station broadcasting twenty-four hours a day and available to an unlimited number of listeners.

Some polyamorists have complained that while love may be unlimited, time appears finite, but I've noticed that time often seems to expand when I stop telling myself there's not enough of it. For now, let's just notice how a situation in which love is shared among several partners is going to be painful if we're holding the belief that love is like a pie and pleasurable if we think of it as an experience that is enhanced when others also enjoy it.

Another of the natural laws of love that polyamory inevitably highlights is the *law of unity*. Simply stated, in the new paradigm, we realize that love knows no borders and no boundaries. Love includes everyone and everything. It takes no position and rises above separation. This doesn't mean that discernment about how and when to express love goes out the window, nor does it mean that the expression of love automatically involves sex. Instead, this new-paradigm law offers a context in which the reality of Oneness can be embodied, and practical, mutually agreeable strategies for inclusion can be negotiated with a partner or partners instead of reacting with guilt, shame, and blame.

The old paradigm for love enshrined jealousy and possessiveness. Instead of discouraging jealousy and possessiveness so that people could freely choose how they would mate, the old paradigm for love established cultural and moral barriers intended to eliminate legitimate alternatives. By drawing a line around the couple or the nuclear family and saying, in effect, "inside this circle we share love and selflessly look out for each other, but outside this circle we keep anyone and everyone from taking what is ours," an illusion of artificial boundaries that is increasingly difficult to maintain was created.

Altruism is another expression of the law of unity. It refers to the choice to unselfishly do something that benefits someone else even to one's own apparent detriment because the illusion of separation has been replaced with the new-paradigm reality that we are all part of the same whole. While many people willingly embrace altruism when it comes to their children or even strangers, one of the greatest challenges to experiencing joy and generosity in someone else's good fortune seems to arise where sharing erotic or romantic love is involved. The word *compersion* grew out of the experience of polyamorous people in the Kerista commune who noticed that it was far more enjoyable to enthusiastically accept the love and pleasure their partners found with each other than to resist it.

We need not rely on logic to decide whether separation is an illusion. If we turn instead to our direct experience, it soon becomes apparent that while the skin is a kind of physical container for the body, we are able to sense activity beyond the boundaries of the physical body. More dramatically, without a constant intake of oxygen from "outside," life on the "inside" soon ceases. Science now tells us that the same molecules that make up our bodies are rapidly recycled and exchanged with other entities. The same, of course, is true for the need for resources from outside the boundary of the family. A single individual or a single couple or family cannot exist without ongoing interactions with a larger human and natural environment.

Polyamory breaks down cultural patterns of control as well as ownership and property rights between persons and, by replacing them with a family milieu of unconditional love, trust, and respect, provides an avenue to the creation of a more just and peaceful world. By changing the size, structure, and emotional context of the family, the personalities of the children developing in these families naturally change. Children learn by example. We cannot teach our children to share and to love one another when we jealously guard and covertly control our most precious possessions—our spouses. By making the boundaries of the family more flexible and more permeable to the outside world, we set the stage for a new worldview in which we recognize our kinship with all of humanity.

Polyamory also offers abundant opportunities to practice the *law of forgiveness*. This law is crucial because forgiveness is both the means by which it's possible to love oneself and others unconditionally and the evidence of this love. The nature of being human is that we make mistakes, especially when attempting a new and challenging way of loving. Without always allowing a second chance, this effort would be doomed. It is the capacity to forgive and forget that allows us to release conditional love one condition at a time, as many times as necessary. When someone loves us, even after finding out about our secret "flaws," even knowing that we may love and desire others, the separation we feel from love is healed. This healing is forgiveness.

Shifting our beliefs about love in all these ways directly benefits those involved by creating more functional and workable relationships. At the same time, these effects ripple out as a gift to the rest of the world.

POLYAMORY AS A GROWTH ACCELERATOR

At the start of the sexual revolution in the 1960s, many people thought that creating honest nonmonogamous relationships would be easy. Instead, half a century of false starts and painful discoveries has taught us that polyamory exacts a price. The fact is that most twenty-first-century humans have many contradictory impulses that pull us in the direction of inclusive love and simultaneously push us in the direction of jealousy and possessiveness. These opposing forces must be reconciled before we are truly free to love. Polyamory places people in the center of the cyclone, with an abundance of opportunities to confront these opposing forces and to learn from their mistakes along the way. Learning theorists have found that the more mistakes you make, the faster you learn. In polyamory, it's possible to get the benefit of several lifetimes worth of mistakes in a relatively short time because you are engaging in more than one intimate relationship at a time.

Polyamorous relationships have another major advantage in accelerating personal growth. Intimate relationships at their best are a path to higher consciousness and greater self-knowledge, largely because of the valuable feedback—or mirroring effect—one receives from a beloved. Having more than one partner at a time not only increases the available quantity of feedback but also makes it harder to blame your partner for the problems you might be creating in the relationship. Of course, serial monogamy also offers the opportunity to see the same issues arise in one relationship after another, but not only does it take longer to get the lesson, but, if you're a fast talker, you may be able to convince one person at a time that it's not your fault, whereas two are less likely to be fooled.

Bill is an attractive man in his late forties who has never been married. Over the years, he'd had a series of monogamous relationships, each lasting about four years. "I'm not sure why none of these relationships lasted," he told me. "I always assumed it just wasn't a match and moved on to the next woman, but I'm getting older, and I really want to settle down." Bill decided he wanted to try polyamory and took my advice to start by seeking out women who weren't seeking a monogamous commitment. Soon he was dating three different women and was thrilled when it turned out that two of them knew and liked each other. After a few months, however, he found himself struggling. "Liz, Helen, and Angie are all mad at me," he complained. "They started comparing notes and found out I'd told some white lies. Now they're accusing me of manipulating them. I really don't understand what their problem is, but I'd like to find out. Can you help me?" Bill was reaping the benefits of polyamory in a different way than he'd expected, but his openness to taking a look at himself—once three women instead of one were insisting on it—was promising.

Because multiple-partner relationships are inherently more complex and demanding than monogamous ones and because they challenge the norms of our culture, they offer other valuable learning opportunities. Lessons about loving yourself, about tolerance for diversity, about speaking from the heart and communicating clearly, and about learning to trust an internal sense of rightness and to think for yourself rather than blindly relying on outside opinion are only a sampling of the lessons. These qualities are earmarks of an emotionally and spiritually mature person—the kind of person who makes a good parent and who can contribute to his or her community.

POLYAMORY AND THE FUTURE OF THE FAMILY

One of the most common concerns about polyamory is that it's harmful to children, but nothing could be farther from the truth. As we saw in chapter 7, multiple-adult families and committed intimate networks have the potential of providing dependent children with additional nurturing adults who can meet their material, intellectual, and emotional needs. While parents may end up focusing less attention on their children, children may gain new aunts, uncles, and adopted parents.

More adults sharing parenting can mean less stress and less burnout without losing any of the rewards. In a larger group of men and women, it's more likely that one or two adults will be willing and able to stay home and care for the family or that each could be available one or two days a week. If one parent dies or becomes disabled, other family members can fill the gap. It's possible for children to have more role models, more playmates, and more love in a group environment. Of course, these advantages can be found in any community setting, but people sometimes avoid intimacy with other adults in a conscious or unconscious effort to safeguard a monogamous commitment.

Polyamory can help create stable and nurturing families where children develop in an atmosphere of love and security. With the traditional nuclear family well on its way to extinction, we are faced with a question of critical importance: who will mind the children? Neither two-career nor single-parent families offer children full-time, loving caretakers, and quality day care is both scarce and expensive. Even at its best, full-time institutional care (including public schooling) cannot provide the individual attention, intimacy, flexibility, and opportunity for solitude that children need to realize their potential. Serial monogamy presents children as well as parents with a stressfully discontinuous family life. Meanwhile, an entire generation is at risk, as divorce is an increasingly common fact of life.

We don't yet know how polyamory impacts the rate of divorce; the little data we have suggest that it doesn't. Some people have begun to joke about "serial polyamory," and it may turn out that any kind of lasting relationship is simply less likely in the twenty-first century. We do know that practicing polyamory can help prepare parents to maintain family ties after a divorce because the issue of becoming jealous when confronted with a former mate's new partner has usually been dealt with already.

Polyamory can mean a higher standard of living while consuming fewer resources. Sexualoving partners are more likely than friends or neighbors to feel comfortable sharing housing, transportation, appliances, and other resources. Even if partners don't live communally, they frequently share meals, help each other with household repairs and projects, and vacation together. This kind of cooperation helps provide a higher quality of life while reducing individual consumption as well as keeping people too busy to overconsume. Multiple partners also help in the renewal of our devastated human ecology by creating a sense of bonded community.

Polyamory can help parents and children alike adapt to an ever more complex and quickly changing world. One of the greatest challenges facing humans at the dawn of the twenty-first century is coping with the increasingly fast pace of life. We're constantly being inundated with more information than we can absorb and more choices than we can evaluate. New technologies are becoming obsolete almost before we can implement them. Trying to keep up can be stressful if not impossible for a single person or a couple. But a small group of loving and well-coordinated partners can divide up tasks that would overwhelm one or two people. Multiple-partner relationships can be an antidote to future shock.

POLYAMORY AND CHANGING SEX ROLE STEREOTYPES

One of the most difficult challenges confronting men and women in the twenty-first century is making the transition from the rigid and well-defined gender identities prevalent in the twentieth century to the more fluid and androgynous roles preferred by many individuals. Diverse opinions as to the healthiest, most natural, and most functional approach to gender roles are still being debated by social scientists, psychotherapists, and spiritual teachers. Most people would agree, however, that both John Wayne–style masculinity and the classic 1950s housewife version of femininity, as well as any identity based solely on gender, are prescriptions for unhappiness. While the extreme versions of these old stereotypes are increasingly rare, many people are still struggling with the more subtle effects of generations of gender-based tyranny.

Marriage as we know it today is based on patterns established in biblical times governing men's ownership of women. Polyamory can help men and women break out of dysfunctional sex roles and achieve more equal, sexually gratifying, and respectful relationships simply because of its novelty. Most of us have unconsciously absorbed our culture's messages about proper demeanor for husbands and wives. We may think our modern society has left this legacy behind, but remember that women in the United States have had the right to vote for less than 100 years. Polyamory leads us to confront the sex role conditioning of our ancestors and demands that we transcend it. It requires that men and women alike overcome our competitive programming and that we invent new ways of relating since we can no longer fall back on simply doing it the way Mom and Dad or Grandma and Grandpa did it.

There's no doubt that polyamory presents multiple challenges to those attempting to practice it. The stakes are high when we put our hearts, minds, and bodies on the line, but the reality is that refusing to do so is becoming increasingly untenable.

NOTES

INTRODUCTION

1. Robert Masters, *Transformation through Intimacy* (Surrey, BC: Tehmenos Press, 2007).

2. Edmund Bourne, *Global Shift* (Oakland, CA: New Harbinger, 2009), 2.

CHAPTER 1

1. Sarah Blaffer Hrdy, "The Primate Origins of Human Sexuality," in *The Evolution of Sex*, ed. Robert Bellig and George Stevens (San Francisco: Harper and Row, 1988).

2. Ramana Maharshi, *Forty Verses on Reality*, trans. S. S. Cohen (Tiruvannamalai, India: Sri Ramanasharam, 2008).

3. Theresa Crenshaw, *The Alchemy of Love and Lust* (New York, G. P. Putnam, 1996), 3.

4. Helen Fisher, Lecture at the American Psychiatric Association annual meeting, 2004.

5. Hasse Walum, paper presented at the Proceedings of the National Academy of Sciences, September 1–5, 2008.

6. Marnia Robinson, "The Mysteries of Pair Bonding (Part II)," Psychologytoday.com, November 10, 2009, https://www.psychologytoday.com, November 30, 2009.

CHAPTER 2

1. Nancy Casey, "Polyamory as a Spiritual Partnership," *Loving More*, no. 39, Spring 2010, 23–25.

2. Kamala Devi, e-mail communication, November 17, 2009.

3. Sonia Song, *Donkey Baby: From Beijing to Berkeley and Beyond* (Bloomington, IN: Author House, 2008), 259.

4. C. T. Butler, e-mail communication, December 7, 2009.

5. Amy Marsh, http://carnalnation.com/content/37497/999/road-tantra?page=0,0, November 18, 2009.

6. Amy Marsh, personal communication, November 17, 2009. See also http://www.tantra-intimacy-aspergers.com.

7. Esther Perel, *Mating in Captivity: Unlocking Erotic Intelligence* (New York: Harper, 2007), 198–99.

8. Perel, *Mating in Captivity*, 199.

9. Robert Masters, *Transformation through Intimacy* (Surrey, BC: Tehmenos Press, 2007), 2.

10. Byron Katie, online newsletter.

11. Byron Katie, *Loving What Is* (Three Rivers, CA: Three Rivers Press, 2003).

12. David J. Ley, *Insatiable Wives: Women Who Stray and the Men Who Love Them* (Lanham, MD: Rowman & Littlefield, 2009).

13. David J. Ley, personal communication, November 2009.

14. Ley, *Insatiable Wives*, 113.

15. Dane Colby, *101 Choices on My Path to Well-Being: Choosing Happiness over Normalcy as a Highly Sensitive Person with Aspergers Syndrome*, http://www.lulu.com/content/5582544, 2008.

16. Peter M. Thomas, "Dissociation and Internal Models of Protection: Psychotherapy with Child Abuse Survivors," *Psychotherapy: Theory, Research, Practice, Training* 42, no. 1 (2005): 20–23.

17. Janet Kira Lessin, *Polyamory, Many Loves, the Poly-Tantric Lovestyle: A Personal Account* (Bloomington, IN: Author House, 2006).

18. Jasmine Walston, "Polyamory: An Exploratory Study of Responsible Multi-Partnering," paper presented at the Building Bridges Conference of the Institute for Twenty-First Century Relationships, Seattle, June 2001.

19. Adam Weber, "Survey Results: Who Are We?," *Loving More*, no. 30, Summer 2002, 4–6.

20. Meg Barker, "This Is My Partner, and This Is My Partner's Partner: Constructing Polyamorous Identity in a Monogamous World," *Journal of Constructivist Psychology* 18 (2005): 75–88.

CHAPTER 3

1. Beth Quinn Barnard, "The Utopia of Sharing in Oneida, NY," *New York Times*, August 3, 2007.

2. "Jacob Cochran," *Wikipedia, the Free Encyclopedia*, http://en.wikipedia.org/w/index.php?title=Jacob_Cochran&oldid=302830918, July 18, 2009.

3. J. Beecher and R. Bienvenu, *The Utopian Vision of Charles Fourier* (Boston: Beacon Press, 1971).

4. Emma Goldman, *Living My Life* (New York: Knopf, 1931).

5. Barbara Foster, Michael Foster, and Letha Hadady, *Three in Love* (New York: HarperCollins, 1997).

6. Oberon Zell (personal communication).

7. Oberon Zell (personal communication).

8. Starhawk, *The Fifth Sacred Thing* (New York: Bantam, 1993).

9. Anna Francoeur and Robert Francoeur, *Hot and Cool Sex* (New York: Harcourt Brace Jovanovich, 1974).

10. Raymond Lawrence, *The Poisoning of Eros* (New York: Augustine Moore Press, 1990).

11. Cyra McFadden, *The Serial* (New York: Knopf, 1977).

12. James Ramey, *Intimate Friendships* (Englewood Cliffs, NJ: Prentice Hall, 1976).

13. Ryam Nearing, "I Know You're Experienced, but Are You Responsible?," *Loving More*, Summer 1995, 29.

14. Loraine Hutchins and Lani Kaahumanu, *Bi Any Other Name: Bisexual People Speak Out* (Boston: Alyson Publications, 1991).

15. Brad Blanton, *Radical Honesty* (Stanley, VA: Sparrowhawk Publications, 2005).

CHAPTER 4

1. FM Esfandiary (personal communication).

2. FM Esfandiary, "Intimacy in a Fluid World," *In Context*, Summer 1985, 39, http://www.context.org/ICLIB/IC10/Esfandry.htm (accessed July 20, 2006).

3. Esfandiary, "Intimacy in a Fluid World," 41.

4. Jim Ramey, *Intimate Friendships* (Englewood Cliffs, NJ: Prentice Hall, 1976).

5. Riane Eisler, *Sacred Pleasure: Sex, Myth, and the Politics of the Body* (San Francisco: Harper, 1995).

6. Deborah Anapol, *The Seven Natural Laws of Love* (Santa Rosa, CA: Elite Books, 2005).

7. Carter Heyward, *Touching Our Strength: The Erotic as Power and the Love of God* (San Francisco: HarperCollins, 1995).

8. Rustum Roy and Della Roy, *Honest Sex* (New York: New American Library, 1968).

9. George O'Neill and Nena O'Neill, *Open Marriage* (New York: M. Evans, 1972).

10. Arthur Waskow, "Down to Earth Judaism: Sexuality," http://www.tikkun.org/media-gallery/download.php?mid=20090505112546716 (accessed October 19, 2009).

11. Gershon Winkler, *Sacred Secrets* (Northvale, NJ: Jason Aronson, 1998).

12. Jayaram V, "Polyamory in Hinduism in Theory and Practice," http://www.hinduwebsite.com/hinduism/h_polygamy.asp (accessed October 22, 2009).

13. Osho, *Love, Freedom, and Aloneness* (New York: St. Martin's Press, 2001).

14. Author's unpublished research.

15. Huma Ahmad, "Top Ten Misconceptions about Islam," http://www.jannah.org/articles/misc.html (accessed October 22, 2009).

16. Richard Sutphen, *Radical Spirituality* (Malibu, CA: Valley of the Sun, 1995).

17. Jorge Ferrer, "Monogamy, Polyamory, and Beyond," *Tikkun*, June 2009, http://www.tikkun.org/article.php?story=Ferrer-monogamy-polyamory-and-beyond (accessed October 20, 2009).

18. Byron Katie and Stephen Mitchell, *A Thousand Names for Joy* (New York: Three Rivers Press, 2007).

19. Byron Katie, "The Work on Relationships" (public lecture, Marin County, CA, 2002).

20. Carl Rogers, *Marriage and Its Alternatives* (New York: Delacourte Press, 1972).

21. Bertrand Russell, *Marriage and Morals* (New York: Bantam Books, 1959).

22. Associated Press, "The Governors Secret," http://www.aolcdn.com/ke/media_gallery/v1/ke_media_gallery_wrapper.swf, (accessed October 15, 2009).

23. Werner Erhard, Michael C. Jensen, and Steve Zaffron, "Integrity: A Positive Model That Incorporates the Normative Phenomena of Morality, Ethics, and Legality," http://ssrn.com/abstract=920625 (accessed October 23, 2009).

CHAPTER 5

1. Geri Weitzman, "Therapy with Clients Who Are Bisexual and Polyamorous," *Journal of Bisexuality* 6, no. 1/2 (2006): 137–64.

CHAPTER 6

1. Thomas Moore, *Care of the Soul* (New York: HarperCollins, 1992).

2. Daniel Goleman, *Emotional Intelligence* (New York: Bantam Books, 1995).

3. Gordon Clanton and Lynn G. Smith, eds., *Jealousy* (Englewood Cliffs, NJ: Prentice Hall, 1977).

4. David Buss, *The Dangerous Passion: Why Jealousy Is as Necessary as Sex and Love* (New York: Free Press, 2000).

5. Buss, *The Dangerous Passion*.

6. Elizabeth Gould David, *The First Sex* (Baltimore: Penguin, 1972).

7. E. S. Craghill Handy and Mary Kawena Pukui, *The Polynesian Family System in Ka'u, Hawaii* (Honolulu: Mutual Publishing, 1999).

8. James Slack, "Judges Sink Harriet Harman's 'Obnoxious' Plan to Strip Men of Infidelity Murder Defence," *Daily Mail*, October 28, 2009, http://www.dailymail.co.uk/news/article-1223367/Judges-sink-Harriet-Harmans-obnoxious-plan-strip-men-infidelity-murder-defence.html#ixzz0VkDwiKPH (accessed November 3, 2009).

9. Afua Hirsch, "Murder Law Reform," *Guardian*, January 19, 2009, http://www.guardian.co.uk/uk/2009/jan/19/murder-law-reform-provocation (accessed November 3, 2009).

10. Meredith Small, "What's Love Got to Do with It?" *Discover*, June 1992, 46–51.

CHAPTER 7

1. Samuel Widmer, e-mail, December 1, 2009.

2. Maria Pallotta-Chiarolli, *Border Sexualities, Border Families in Schools* (New York: Rowman & Littlefield, 2010).

3. Maria Pallotta-Chiarolli, "Polyparents, Having Children, Raising Children, Schooling Children," in *Understanding Non-Monogamies*, ed. Meg Barker and Darren Langridge (London: Routledge, 2010).

4. Pallotta-Chiarolli, "Polyparents, Having Children, Raising Children, Schooling Children."

5. Maria Pallotta-Chiarolli, *Love You Two* (North Sydney: Random House, 2008).

6. Larry Constantine and Joan Constantine, *Group Marriage: A Study of Contemporary Multilateral Marriage* (New York: Macmillan, 1973).

7. Elisabeth Sheff, personal communication, November 5, 2009. Dr. Sheff can be contacted via e-mail at soceasx@langate.gsu.edu.

8. Becca Tzigany and J. G. Bertrand, *The Pillow Book of Venus and Her Lover: Reinventing the Myth*, 2009, http://www.venusandherlover.com.

9. Valerie White, "Checklist for Poly Parents," http://www.sfldef.org/Checklist for Poly_Parents.htm (accessed October 23, 2009).

10. Kenn Thomas and Len Bracken, "The Finder's Keeper," Steamshovel Press, #16, 1998, http://www.mail-archive.com/ctrl@listserv.aol.com/msg00344.html (accessed November 30, 2009).

11. Osho, *Love, Freedom, and Aloneness* (New York: St. Martin's Press, 2001), 137–38.

CHAPTER 8

1. Lisa M. Diamond, *Sexual Fluidity: Understanding Women's Love and Desire* (Cambridge, MA: Harvard University Press, 2009).

2. Daniel Cardosa, Carla Correia, and Danielle Capella, "Polyamory as a Possibility of Feminine Empowerment" (paper presented at the Ninth Congress of the European Sociological Association, Lisbon, Portugal, September 2009).

3. Cardosa et al., "Polyamory as a Possibility of Feminine Empowerment," 13–14.

4. Geri Weitzman, "Therapy with Clients Who Are Bisexual and Polyamorous," *Journal of Bisexuality* 6, no. 1–2 (2006): 137–64.

CHAPTER 9

1. Esther Perel, *Mating in Captivity* (New York: Harper, 2007), 55.

2. "Sexual Revolution Silently Going On in China," *Xinhua Online*, http://news.xinhuanet.com/english/2005-06/03/content_3041598.htm (accessed November 22, 2009).

3. Sonia Song, *Donkey Baby* (Bloomington, IN: Authorhouse, 2008), 259.

4. Dossie Easton (personal communication and unpublished paper, October 2009).

5. Leila Dregger, "Project Meiga: How It All Began," in *Liberating Love: Readings from the German Meiga Communities*, trans. Eva Langrock, ed. Jock Millenson (Forres, Scotland: Juggler Press, 2007), 11.

6. Alan MacRoberts, "Seven Poly Books Upcoming," *Polyamory in the News*, http://polyinthemedia.blogspot.com/2009/12/xx-new-poly-books-in-works.html (accessed December 6, 2009).

7. Samuel Widmer, http://www.samuel-widmer.ch (accessed September 18, 2009).

8. Komaja Community, "Manifesto for Polyamory," http://www.komaja.org/en/polyamory_manifest.php, 2006 (accessed November 18, 2009).

9. Serena Anderlini D'Onofrio, "Midsummer Dreams in New Central Europe: Meeting the Komaja Community," *Loving More*, Spring 2007, 12–14.

10. Dossie Easton and Janet Hardy, *The Ethical Slut: Polyamory, Open Relationships and Other Adventures* (2nd ed.) (Berkeley, CA: Ten Speed Press, 2009).

11. Dossie Easton (unpublished paper, October 2009).

12. Meg Barker and Darren Langridge, eds., *Understanding Non-Monogamies* (London: Routledge, 2009).

13. Meg Barker (personal communication, 2009).

14. Andie Nordgren, http://andie.se, November 2009.

15. Deborah Anapol, *Polyamory: The New Love without Limits* (San Rafael, CA: Intinet, 1997), 5.

16. Maria Palloti-Chiarolli, "Polyparents, Having Children, Raising Children, Schooling Children," in *Understanding Non-Monogamies*, ed. Meg Barker and Darren Langridge (London: Routledge, 2009), 182–87.

17. Petula Sik Ying Ho, "The Charmed Circle Game: Reflections on Sexual Hierarchy through Multiple Sexual Relationships," *Sexualities* 9 (2006): 547.

CHAPTER 10

1. Elizabeth Gilbert, *Eat, Pray, Love* (New York: Penguin, 2006), 149.

2. Robert Graves and Raphael Patai, *Hebrew Myths: The Book of Genesis* (New York: Doubleday, 1964).

3. Barbara Foster, Michael Foster, and Letha Hadady, *Three in Love* (San Francisco: HarperCollins, 1997).

4. Doug Slinger and Penny Slinger, *Sexual Secrets* (New York: Destiny Books, 1979).

5. Muna Tseng, "Ming Fei," in *The Union of Sex and Spirit*, ed. Mary de G. White (New York: Cauldron Productions, 1993).

6. Merlin Stone, *When God Was a Woman* (New York: Harcourt Brace Jovanovich, 1976).

7. Andie Norgren (e-mail communication, December 3, 2009).

8. David Barash and Judith Lipton, *The Myth of Monogamy* (New York: W. H. Freeman, 2001).

9. Leslie Temple Thurston, *Marriage of Spirit* (Santa Fe, NM: CoreLight Publications, 2000).

10. Gina Haddon, *Uniting Sex, Self, and Spirit* (Scotland, CT: Plus Publications, 1993).

11. Jean Shinoda Bolen, *Goddesses in Every Woman* (San Francisco: Harper & Row, 1984).

12. Nikolaos A. Vrissimtzis, *Love, Sex, and Marriage in Ancient Greece* (Athens: Polygrama, 1997).

13. Verrier Elwin, http://www.purpleonion.nl/background/bastar (accessed November 1, 2009).

14. E. S. Graghill Handy and Mary Kawena Pukui, *The Polynesian Family System in Ka'u, Hawaii* (Honolulu: Mutual Publishing, 1998).

15. Lynn Margulis and Dorion Sagan, *Mystery Dance: On the Evolution of Human Sexuality* (New York: Summit Books, 1991).

16. Margulis and Sagan, *Mystery Dance*.

17. Sarah Blaffer Hrdy, "The Primate Origins of Human Sexuality," in *The Evolution of Sex*, ed. Robert Bellig and George Stevens (San Francisco: Harper & Row, 1988).

18. Meredith Small, "What's Love Got to Do with It?," *Discover*, June 1992, 46–51.

19. Ken Wilber, *The Atman Project* (Wheaton, IL: Theosophical Publishing House, 1980).

20. Spider Robinson and Jeanne Robinson, *Stardance* (New York: Dial Press, 1979).

21. Pierre Teilhard de Chardin, *The Future of Man* (New York: Harper Colophon, 1969).

22. Dane Rudhyar, *Directives for New Life* (Rail Road Flat, CA: Seed Publications, 1971).

CHAPTER 11

1. A. Pawlowski, "Mate Debate: Is Monogamy Realistic?," *CNN.com*, http://www.cnn.com/2009/LIVING/10/28/monogamy.realistic.today/index.html (accessed November 1, 2009).

2. Serena Anderlini-D'Onofrio, *Gaia and the New Politics of Love: Notes for a Poly Planet* (Berkeley, CA: North Atlantic Books, 2009).

3. James Lovelock, *Gaia: A New Look at Life on Earth* (Oxford: Oxford University Press, 1979).

4. Anderlini-D'Onofrio, *Gaia and the New Politics of Love*, 41.

5. Anderlini-D'Onofrio, *Gaia and the New Politics of Love*, 5.

6. Anderlini-D'Onofrio, *Gaia and the New Politics of Love*, 115.

7. Anderlini-D'Onofrio, *Gaia and the New Politics of Love*, 137.

8. James W. Prescott, "Body Pleasure and the Origins of Violence," *Bulletin of the Atomic Scientists*, November 1975, 10–20.

9. Prescott, "Body Pleasure and the Origins of Violence."

10. Dolores LaChappelle, *Sacred Land, Sacred Sex: Rapture of the Deep* (Durango, CO: Kivaki Press, 1988).

11. LaChappelle, *Sacred Land, Sacred Sex*, 260.
12. LaChappelle, *Sacred Land, Sacred Sex*, 261.
13. LaChappelle, *Sacred Land, Sacred Sex*, 263.
14. Deborah Anapol, *The Seven Natural Laws of Love* (Santa Rosa, CA: Elite Books, 2005).

SELECTED BIBLIOGRAPHY

Anapol, Deborah. *Polyamory: The New Love without Limits*. San Rafael, CA: Intinet, 1997.

——. *The Seven Natural Laws of Love*. Santa Rosa, CA: Elite Books, 2005.

Anderlini-D'Onofrio, Serena. *Gaia and the New Politics of Love: Notes for a Poly Planet*. Berkeley, CA: North Atlantic Books, 2009.

Barash, David, and Judith Lipton *The Myth of Monogamy*. New York: W. H. Freeman, 2001.

Barker, Meg, and Darren Langridge, eds. *Understanding Non-Monogamies*. London: Routledge, 2009.

Blanton, Brad, *Radical Honesty*. Stanley, VA: Sparrowhawk Publications, 2005.

Campbell, Susan. *Truth in Dating*. Tiburon, CA: New World Library, 2004.

Diamond, Lisa M. *Sexual Fluidity: Understanding Women's Love and Desire*, Cambridge, MA: Harvard University Press, 2009.

Easton, Dossie, and Janet Hardy. *The Ethical Slut: Polyamory, Open Relationships and Other Adventures*. 2nd ed. Berkeley, CA: Ten Speed Press, 2009.

Eisler, Riane. *Sacred Pleasure: Sex, Myth, and the Politics of the Body*. San Francisco: Harper, 1995.

Fisher, Helen. *The Anatomy of Love*. New York: Norton, 1992.

Foster, Barbara, Michael Foster, and Letha Hadady. *Three in Love*. San Francisco: HarperCollins, 1997.

Francoeur, Anna, and Robert Francoeur. *Hot and Cool Sex*. New York: Harcourt Brace Jovanovich, 1974.

Goldman, Emma. *Living My Life*. New York: Knopf, 1931.

Heyward, Carter. *Touching Our Strength: The Erotic as Power and the Love of God*. San Francisco: HarperCollins, 1995.

Hutchins, Loraine, and Lani Kaahumanu. *Bi Any Other Name: Bisexual People Speak Out*. Boston: Alyson Publications, 1991.

Katie, Byron. *Loving What Is*. Three Rivers, CA: Three Rivers Press, 2003.

LaChappelle, Dolores. *Sacred Land, Sacred Sex: Rapture of the Deep*. Durango, CO: Kivaki Press, 1988.

Ley, David J. *Insatiable Wives: Women Who Stray and the Men Who Love Them*. Lanham, MD: Rowman & Littlefield, 2009.

Margulis, Lynn, and Dorion Sagan. *Mystery Dance: On the Evolution of Human Sexuality*. New York: Summit Books, 1991.

Masters, Robert. *Transformation through Intimacy*. Surrey, BC: Tehmenos Press, 2007.

Mazur, Ronald. *The New Intimacy*. Lincoln, NE: toExcel, 2000.

Ogden, Gina. *The Return of Desire*. Boston: Trumpeter Books, 2008.

O'Neill, George, and Nena O'Neill. *Open Marriage*. New York: M. Evans, 1972.

Osho. *Love, Freedom, and Aloneness*. New York: St. Martin's Press, 2001.

Pallotta-Chiarolli, Maria. *Border Sexualities, Border Families in Schools*. New York: Rowman & Littlefield, 2009.

Perel, Esther. *Mating in Captivity*. New York: Harper, 2007.

Ramey, James. *Intimate Friendships*. Englewood Cliffs, NJ: Prentice Hall, 1976.

Rimmer, Robert. *The Harrad Experiment*. Buffalo, NY: Prometheus Books, 1990.

Rogers, Carl. *Marriage and Its Alternatives*. New York: Delacourte Press, 1972.

Russell, Bertrand. *Marriage and Morals*. New York: Bantam Books, 1959.

Roy, Rustum, and Della Roy. *Honest Sex*. New York: New American Library, 1968.

Song, Sonia. *Donkey Baby*. Bloomington, IN: Authorhouse, 2008.

Starhawk. *The Fifth Sacred Thing*. New York: Bantam, 1993.

Taormino, Tristan. *Opening Up*. San Francisco: Cleis Press, 2008.

Winkler, Gershon. *Sacred Secrets*. Northvale, NJ: Jason Aronson, 1998.

INDEX

acceptance as new-paradigm value, 68, 133

accountability, 103

activists/activism, 23, 25–26, 53, 173, 181, 197; gay, lesbian, bisexual, transgendered, and queer (GLBTQ), 61–62, 204

adolescents: perspectives and experiences of, 92, 93, 97, 132–33, 135–40, 150–53, 171–72; polyamory as challenging for, 138–39. *See also* children

adultery: biblical prohibition against, 67; Judaism and, 71–72. *See also* affairs; infidelity

affairs, extramarital: common in cultures espousing monogamy, 5, 7, 12–13; case material, 38, 87, 109–10, 115, 208–9; European relaxed attitude toward, 185; jealousy and, 109, 113, 115; media portrayals of, 141; politicians and exposure of, 77, 231–32. *See also* extramarital sex; infidelity; jealousy

agreements: commitment and, 13; decision making and, 78–80; integrity as essential to, 80–81; new sexual ethic and, 78–80

Akbar, Jalaluddin Muhammad (emperor), 73

alpha behavior, 9

"alpha problem," 103–4

altruism, 9–10, 237, 239

anarchist politics, 24–26, 207

anarchy, relationship. *See* relationship anarchy

Anderlini-D'Onofrio, Serena, 203, 233–36

androgen, 11

animals: mating patterns in, 6–10, 113–14, 213; pleasure and violence in, 235–36. *See also* primates

Aphrodite, 221

archetypes, 213–14, 219–22. *See also* mythology

response to, in men *vs.* women, 106; overcoming, 113; parental triangle and, 119–21; power struggle and, 124; self-awareness and, 123; as single phenomenon with many triggers, 116; somatic experience/discomfort of, 105, 107–8, 116; spiritual dimension of, 122; systematic desensitization and, 125–26; triggers of, 116–19. *See also* competition; infidelity
Jud, Gerald, 54, 55
Judaism, contemporary, 71–72

Katie, Byron, 38–40, 75
Kennedy, Jivana, 152–53
Kerista Village, 57–58, 153
Khajuraho, India, temple art of, 73, 191, 192
Kirkridge Conferences, 53, 54, 55
Komaja community, 202–3
Kramer, Joseph, 62

LaChapelle, Dolores, 236
law, polyamory and the, 178–82; "dyadic networks" *vs.* "all-with-all" marital legislation, 181–82; India's Hindu Marriage Act, 191; Muslim arguments for plural marriage, 73, 178–79; poly community opinions on legalization, 180–81; renegade Mormons and case in Canada, 179–80
legal issues, 178–82, 191
Lesbian Polyfidelity (West), 61
lesbians. *See* gay, lesbian, bisexual, transgendered, and queer (GLBTQ) people
Lessin, Alex, 42
Lessin, Janet, 42
Lesvos (Lesbos), Greece, 183–84

Ley, David, 40, 41
Lichtenfels, Sabine, 200
line marriage, 57
Linssen, Leonie, 201
Lipton, Judith Eve, 7–9, 230
Li Yin He, 189
love, 234; allowed to expand without expectations, 1; brain and, 10–12; future of, 226–27; honesty and, 62–63; laws of, 238–40; new paradigm for, 5–6, 237–40; relationship form and, ix–x, 4, 5; sex and, xii; sex and educating children about, 134–36, 141–43, 146–47, 151–53; Sonia Song on, 190. *See also* paradigm shift
love addiction. *See* sex and love addiction
Lovelock, James, 233
Love Unlimited: The Joys and Challenges of Open Relationship (Linssen and Wik), 201
Love You Two (Pallotta-Chiarolli), 131
Loving More Conferences, 60
Loving More magazine, 53, 59, 59–61, 60, 61; polyamory survey in 1990s, 43–44
loyalty, 68–69

Mahabharata, 73; polyandry in, 218
"mainstream polyamory" *vs.* relationship anarchy, 206–7
Makaja, 203
Mali, Raj, 194
Margulis, Lynn, 223, 233
Marriage: complex, 45–47; line, 57; Muslim arguments for plural, 73, 178–79; same-gender, 181; traditional, as floundering, 2. *See also* group marriage; open marriage/ open relationship; *specific topics*

ABOUT THE AUTHOR

Deborah Anapol attended Barnard College, graduated Phi Beta Kappa from the University of California at Berkeley, and received her PhD in clinical psychology from the University of Washington in 1981.

Dr. Anapol is a relationship coach who has specialized in working with people exploring polyamory and conscious relating for nearly three decades. She leads seminars internationally and is an entertaining and controversial speaker who has appeared on radio and television programs all across the United States and Canada. She has raised two daughters and has two grandchildren. Visit her in cyberspace at www.lovewithoutlimits.com.